Gynecology
Clinics Illustrated

Gynecology
Clinics Illustrated

Sun Kuie Tay

Singapore General Hospital, Singapore

World Scientific

NEW JERSEY · LONDON · SINGAPORE · BEIJING · SHANGHAI · HONG KONG · TAIPEI · CHENNAI · TOKYO

Published by

World Scientific Publishing Co. Pte. Ltd.
5 Toh Tuck Link, Singapore 596224
USA office: 27 Warren Street, Suite 401-402, Hackensack, NJ 07601
UK office: 57 Shelton Street, Covent Garden, London WC2H 9HE

Library of Congress Cataloging-in-Publication Data
Names: Tay, Sun Kuie, 1954–   author.
Title: Gynecology clinics illustrated / Sun Kuie Tay.
Description: New Jersey : World Scientific, 2018. | Includes index.
Identifiers: LCCN 2017057651| ISBN 9789813229037 (hardcover : alk. paper) |
    ISBN 9813229039 (hardcover : alk. paper)
Subjects: | MESH: Genital Diseases, Female | Case Reports
Classification: LCC RG121 | NLM WP 140 | DDC 618.1--dc23
LC record available at https://lccn.loc.gov/2017057651

British Library Cataloguing-in-Publication Data
A catalogue record for this book is available from the British Library.

For any available supplementary material, please visit
http://www.worldscientific.com/worldscibooks/10.1142/10682#t=suppl

PREFACE

I cannot emphasize more that attendance at clinics physically is a core learning process of clinical medicine. However, clinical teaching of gynecology is facing immense challenge from shortened curriculum time and reduced access of learners to gynecologic patients. This book, which targets clinical students, residents in gynecology, family physicians and nurses, takes a "mentor- apprentice" approach of learning by discussing 23 clinical scenarios which cover the most common gynecologic complaints.

Each clinical scenario is presented in the form of a short statement of the patient's main complaint. The learning objectives are presented in the form of direct questions following the statement. Residents in gynecology and family physicians who have some experience in gynecology are recommended to evaluate their existing knowledge on the subject before reading the detailed information provided in the answer section on the case. Conditions that are related to the complaints and relevant investigations are presented and illustrated with a wide range of clinical photographs to simulate a day-to-day experience in gynecology clinics. The most important diseases relevant to the presenting symptoms are described in detail to reduce the immediate need of the readers to seek larger textbooks for cross references.

By assimilating information on specific clinical problems, this book is distinctly different from traditional textbooks in which information is fragmented in anatomical systems and pathology compartments. This book, however, does not replace the role of traditional textbooks of gynecology for comprehensive details in some diseases.

This book is fully indexed. Readers can refer to this section for a rapid access to information on subjects of interest.

The preparation of this book drew on the author's clinical experience in gynecology of more than three decades. The content includes both the commonly encountered diseases as well as rare conditions of intellectual interests that are relevant to clinical practice. Regardless of the depth of involvement of gynecology care that an individual reader may render to women, the book provides guidance on the approach to diagnosis, investigation and management of specific clinical entities. It also raises the reader's awareness of issues of concern in women's health in general.

I am indebted to my mentors, colleagues in obstetrics and gynecology, pathology, and surgery, and numerous residents, students and nurses who have taught me, enriched my experience in obstetrics and gynecology, and advanced my care of women in need. I, in particular, wish to thank emeritus Professor Albert Singer PhD, DPhil, FRCOG of University College London, UK for being a great mentor and intellectual inspiration to me. Thanks are also extended to my wife and family. Without their sacrifices and endurance, generous and tireless supports and encouragement, I would not have been able to achieve my professional endeavors and the preparation of this book.

Sun Kuie Tay MBBS, MD FRCOG,
Singapore 2017

CONTENTS

CASE 1 — PRIMARY AMENORRHEA

A 16-year-old girl complains that she has yet to experience menstruation.

- Is this abnormal?
- What produces menstruation?
- What conditions may explain her complaint?
- What investigations should be performed on her?

Is This Abnormal?

The onset of puberty in girls is marked by the beginning of ovarian function in estrogen secretion followed by physical development of breast buds detectable as firm nodules directly beneath the nipples. This occurs between the ages of 10 and 11.5 years old and is known as thelarche. The first menstruation, or menarche, should occur within three years of thelarche.

The mean age of menarche is 12.5 years old. Fewer than 10% of girls menstruate before 11 years old and 90% of girls are menstruating by 13.7 years old. Absence of menarche three years after thelarche or after 16 years old is an abnormal delay known as primary amenorrhea.

The incidence of primary amenorrhea is less than 1%.

What Produces Menstruation?

Menstruation is a cyclic uterine bleeding from necrosis and sloughing of functional layer of endometrium. Normal menstruation lasts between 3 and 8 days with an average blood loss of 30 mL in total.

Endometrium is made up of a basal layer and a functional layer composed of glandular endometrial epithelium and stroma. Endometrium draws blood supply from spiral arterioles which are formed by branching of uterine basal and radiate arterioles. During the proliferative phase (day-4 to day-14 of menstrual cycle), estrogen increases the epithelial and stromal cell proliferation with formation and elongation of epithelial glands. The endometrial thickness increases from 2 mm to 8 mm, together with an extension of spiral arterioles into the stroma. During the secretory phase (day-15 to day-28 of menstrual cycle), progesterone restricts mitotic activities and induces gland enlargement and accumulation of glycogen-rich cytoplasmic vacuoles in the epithelial cells. The stromal becomes edematous.

Menstrual phase (day-1 to day-7) is induced by progesterone withdrawal. Just before menstruation, the endometrium is infiltrated with leucocytes with an increase in tissue levels of prostaglandins, thromboxin and endothelin. These vasoactive cytokines mediate spiral arteriole constriction which leads to necrosis and sloughing of the functional layer of endometrium. This is followed by arteriolar relaxation, bleeding and tissue breakdown which form menstruation.

What Conditions may Explain her Complaint?

Primary amenorrhea may result from anatomical, biochemical, or chromosomal abnormalities, or as a consequence of iatrogenic interventions. Conditions causing primary amenorrhea are best understood using a classification based on anatomical location of pathology:

(i) Absence of End Organs

- Müllerian dysgenesis (Mayer-Rokitansky-Kuster-Hauser syndrome: hypoplastic uterus and upper two thirds of vagina)

- Testicular feminization syndrome
- 5-alpha reductase type-2 deficiency

Testicular feminization syndrome is also known as complete androgen insensitive syndrome. This is an X-linked recessive disorder with mutation of androgen receptor genes located in the long arm of X-chromosome. Despite normal 46 XY chromosomal constitution, the loss of functional androgen receptors in the cell surface leads to failure of masculinization of external genitalia in these individuals. Consequently, they develop a normal female phenotype with normal labia, clitoris and vaginal introitus. However, they have normal testes with normal testosterone production and conversion to dihydrotestosterone. The normal secretion of Müllerian-inhibiting factors leads to absence of fallopian tubes, uterus and proximal vagina.

5-alpha reductase type-2 deficiency is an autosomal recessive condition in which the enzyme deficiency leads to failure of conversion of testosterone to biologically active dihydrotestoterone. These cases present with gender ambiguity in the neonatal period. There is, however, absence of fallopian tubes, uterus and vagina. In cases showing phenotypically female external genitalia, the diagnosis may be delayed until puberty when they present with primary amenorrhea.

(ii) Ovarian Dysfunction

- Gonadal dysgenesis (Turner syndrome)
- Spontaneous 46XX primary ovarian insufficiency
- Autoimmune oophoritis
- Iatrogenic causes: e.g. radiation or chemotherapy.

Turner syndrome was first described by Henry Turner in 1938 for girls with 45XO karyotype. Since then, other chromosomal aberrations have been described, in particular, isochromosome i(Xp) or i(Xq). The classical 45XO accounts for only 50% of Turner syndrome today. The incidence of Turner syndrome is approximately 1 in 2000 female live births. The diagnosis is made at birth in 15%, during childhood in 20%, at teen ages in 25%, and in adulthood in 40%. The most common presenting features are short stature, web neck, increased cubitus valgus, failure to develop puberty, primary amenorrhea from ovarian agenesis or secondary amenorrhea from ovarian dysgenesis or premature failure, infertility, and other endocrinopathy, cardiovascular disorders and osteoporosis. The primary treatment of Turner syndrome is targeted at puberty development with combination of growth hormone and estrogen, and estrogen replacement therapy during adulthood. The other aspects of treatment are aimed to optimize control of endocrine, cardiovascular and metabolic complications.

(iii) Pituitary Disorders

- Pituitary radiation
- Panhypopituitarism.

(iv) Hypothalamic Disorders

Organic causes:

- Craniopharyngioma or teratoma
- Kallmann syndrome (anosmic hypogonadotrophic hypogonadism — failure to achieve puberty).

Functional causes:

- Anorexia/bulimia
- Extreme obesity
- Chronic disease
- Weight loss
- Malnutrition
- Extreme physical exercise
- Severe stress
- Depression
- Psychotropic drug therapy
- Recreational drug abuse.

(v) Lower Genital Tract Anomaly

- Imperforated hymen
- Vaginal agenesis.

Developmental malformation in the lower genital tract is rare. The estimated incidence ranges from 1 in 4,000 to 1 in 10,000. In these cases, menstruation is formed normally but is concealed by blockade in the lower genital tract, a phenomenon known as cryptomenorhea (concealed menstruation). There may be monthly abdominal pain and the hematomatra and hematocolpos may present as a palpable abdomino-pelvic mass or a pelvic mass on rectal examination. In the case of imperforated hymen, a bluish bulge may be seen at the introitus on physical examination.

(vi) Congenital Adrenal Hyperplasia (CAH)

CAH is encountered in 2% of women with androgen excess. In this condition, 21-hydroxylase deficiency blocks biosynthesis of cortisol and leads to an increased ACTH secretion and excessive adrenal androgen production. CAH is more often seen in primary amenorrhea and in girls with gender ambiguity from the effect of virilization. Rarely, late onset CAH can present as secondary amenorrhea.

What Investigations should be Performed on her?

Primary amenorrhea is a symptom, not a diagnosis. Investigations are critical to reach a diagnosis of the underlying condition leading to amenorrhea. Obtaining a detailed medical history and a thorough physical examination are of paramount importance before deciding on the laboratory tests.

(i) Medical History

A detailed history is mandatory. Neonatal investigation for gender ambiguity, undescended gonads or inguinal herniorrhaphy may suggest gonadal dysgenesis or androgen insensitive syndrome. Cyclic abdominal pain after the age of puberty is suggestive of cryptomenorrhea. There may be a history of endocrinopathy or significant medical conditions and therapy.

(ii) Physical Examination

- Short stature and dysmorphic features may suggest Turner syndrome.
- Absence of breast buds may indicate delayed puberty.
- Abdominal mass may indicate uterine enlargement from cryptomenorrhea or ovarian tumor from ovarian dysgenesis.
- Genital tract anomaly of imperforated hymen may present as a bluish bulge in the introitus. In cases of vaginal atresia, absence of the vagina is clinically evident.
- Clitoromegaly is a sign of virilization from androgen excess.
- Absence of uterus may indicate Müllerian dysgenesis or androgen insensitive syndrome.

(iii) Laboratory Investigations

- Pelvic ultrasound scan is diagnostic of anomaly in the Müllerian system and for detection of hematocorpus.
- High serum FSH/LH levels indicate gonado-dysgenesis or Turner syndrome. Normal FSH/LH levels are consistent with Müllerian dysgenesis or androgen insensitive syndrome.
- Specific investigations may be indicated based on clinical suspicion of the diagnosis, including chromosome analysis, serum cortisol level and androgen levels, and imaging study of the central nervous system.

Key Note

Devoid of a function, menstruation reflects the normal physiology of a woman.

Illustration of Some Conditions that can Cause Primary Amenorrhea

The clinical details of this 20-year-old woman who had never experienced a menstruation showed a well and fit woman at 1.5 m in height and 45 kg in weight. There was no dysmorphic feature. The breast development was Tanner state-4 and pubic hair was absent. The external genitalia was infantile. A pelvic ultrasound showed a small uterus measuring 4.8 cm × 1.4 cm × 2.4 cm. The endometrium was poorly visualized. Both ovaries were small, measuring 1.5 cm × 0.9 cm × 1.8 cm on the right and 1.4 cm × 1.3 cm × 0.5 cm on the left. The serum hormonal profile as shown in the table (below) was consistent with primary ovarian insufficiency. Chromosome analysis showed a balanced X-autosome translocation with breakpoints at Xq21 and 8q24 (marked by the black arrows). The most common phenotype of this chromosomal constitution is premature ovarian insufficiency or primary amenorrhea from gonadal agenesis.

Investigation	Result	Normal Range
FSH	154.3	3–20 mIU/mL (follicular phase)
LH	39.8	2–15 mIU/mL (follicular phase)
Estradiol	<43	9–221 pg/mL (follicular phase)
Progesterone	0.9	0.1–1.5 ng/mL (follicular phase)
Free testosterone	1.7	0.07–13.5 pmol/L
DHEA-SO4	4.13	0.9–11.2 umol/L
Prolactin	10.1	0.5–18.1 ng/mL
Thyroid stimulation hormone	0.62	0.45–6.20 mIU/mL
Chromosome karyotyping	46, X,t (X;8) (q21; q24.2–24.3)	

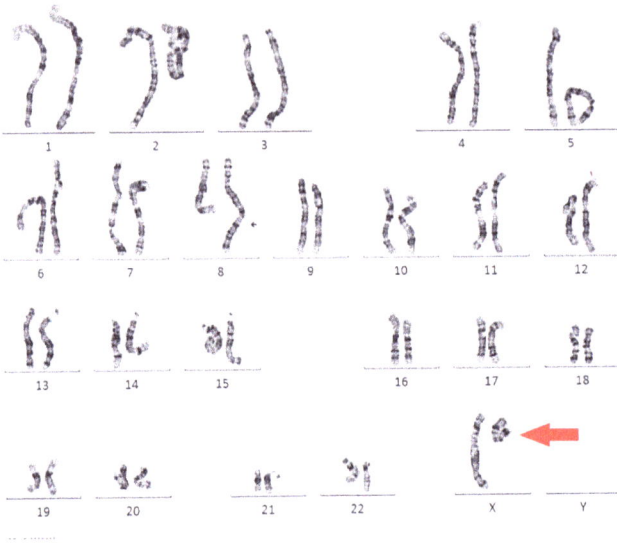

Chromosomal translocation.

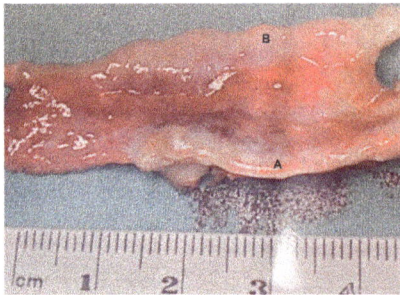

This photograph shows a streak-like ovary in ovarian dysgenesis (A) and a normal fallopian tube (B). This 17-year-old girl, who complained of primary amenorrhea, was found to have a 16-cm immature teratoma in the right ovary and a left streak ovary. Ovarian dysgenesis is associated with a high incidence of malignancy.

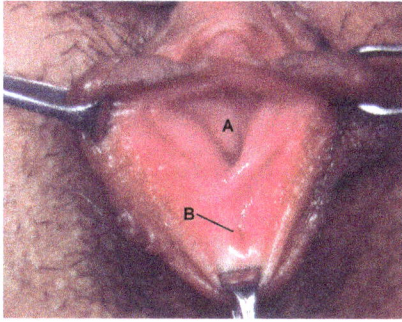

This 20-year-old woman had been married for a year and was investigated for abdominal pain and primary amenorrhea. This photograph shows a dilated urethral meatus (A) through which sexual intercourse occurred. The small dimple inferior to the urethral meatus (B) marked the site of the atretic vagina. Her cryptomenorrhea was successfully corrected with a vaginoplasty procedure.

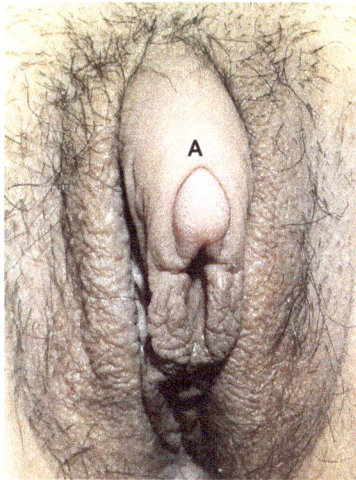

This photograph illustrates an enlarged clitoris (clitoromegaly) marked (A). The normal diameter of clitoris measures 4 mm.

CASE 2 — OLIGO-MENORRHEA

A 25-year-old woman complains of irregular and delayed menstruations for up to three months.

- What is the medical term used to describe her symptom?
- How is the normal menstruation regulated?
- What conditions can cause her symptom?
- What investigations are helpful in achieving a definitive diagnosis?

What is the Medical Term used to Describe her Symptom?

Oligomenorrhea is the term used to define a reduced frequency of menstruation to a cycle length of between 6 weeks and 6 months.

How is the Normal Menstruation Regulated?

Menstruation cycle is regulated via the hypothalamus-pituitary-ovarian-endometrial axis. The pulsatile hypothalamus gonadotrophin releasing hormone (GnRH) stimulates the gonadotrope cells in the anterior pituitary gland to synthesize and release follicle stimulating hormone (FSH) and luteinizing hormone (LH). FSH is critical for ovarian follicle development and maturation, and synthesis of estrogen by the granulosa cells. The follicular phase takes approximately 14 days during which the rising level of circulating estrogen stimulates the proliferation of endometrial epithelial and stroma cells with a resultant thickening of endometrium to 8 mm.

Meanwhile, the elevated serum level of estrogen provides a negative feedback to the pituitary with a switch from FSH to LH secretion. After LH surge and ovulation, the follicle forms corpus luteum which secretes progesterone. Normal luteal phase lasts 14 days during which the progesterone restricts mitotic activity in the epithelial and stromal cells, stimulates endometrial gland enlargement, and induces decidualization of the stroma with marked extension of spiral arteriole into the stroma and extensive entwinement of the arterioles with the glands. In the absence of the stimulatory effect of human chorionic gonadotrophin (HCG) of pregnancy, the corpus luteum regresses (luteolysis). Progesterone withdrawal is accompanied by changes in the endometrial tissue prostaglandin F2α, thromboxin and endothelin secretion. These tissue chemo-mediators induce the constriction of the spiral arterioles. The necrosis and sloughing of the functional layer of endometrium culminate in arteriolar damage, bleeding and tissue breakdown to form menstruation.

The average menstrual cycle lasts 28 days, ranging from 21 to 35 days.

What Conditions can Cause her Symptom?

- Polycystic ovarian syndrome (PCOS)
- Hyperprolactinemia
- Thyroid disorders
- Late onset congenital adrenal hyperplasia
- Cushing syndrome
- Acromegaly
- Lactation
- Menopausal transition
- Weight changes
- Extreme physical exercises
- Psychological/emotional stresses
- Iatrogenic causes: psychotropic medications; progestogen-only contraception.

What Investigations are Helpful in Achieving a Definitive Diagnosis?

(i) Serum FSH, LH and Estradiol profile performed on day-2 of menstruation cycle is useful when a raised serum FSH and LH level is indicative of ovarian failure or resistance. On the other hand, a LH/FSH ratio of >2.5 is indicative of PCOS.

(ii) Serum DHEAS and free testosterone levels: hyperandrogenism may be associated with the classical polycystic ovarian disease also known as the Stein-Leventhal syndrome. Hyperandrogenism may be ovarian or adrenal in origin.

(iii) Serum prolactin level: Elevated serum prolactin level may result from prolactinoma, hypothyroidism, or psychotropic drug induced changes.

(iv) Serum TSH and free T4 levels: primary hypothyroidism is associated with raised hypothalamic thyroid releasing hormone (TRH) secretion. The alpha subunit of TRH may increase prolactin secretion.

(v) Serum 17-hydroxyprogesterone level: a level of less than 1000 ng/dL after a cosyntropin stimulation test rules out late-onset congenital adrenal hyperplasia.

(vi) Serum cortisol and growth hormone is diagnostic for Cushing syndrome and acromegaly.

(vii) Pelvic ultrasound scan: morphological features of the ovaries are diagnostic for PCOS.

Selected Disease

Polycystic ovarian syndrome (PCOS)

PCOS occurs in 4–12% of women in reproductive life. It is seen in 90% of women with oligomenorrhea and 30% of women with secondary amenorrhea. Stein and Leventhal first described in 1935 a group of women characterized by secondary amenorrhea or oligomenorrhea, hirsutism, subfertility, and enlarged ovaries. The defect was thought to be a primary ovarian disease as the capsule of the ovary was thickened and avascular, and there were multiple subcapsular cysts from follicles at various stages of atresia.

Histologically, there was hyperplasia of theca stroma and theca cell luteinization. Today, this disorder is seen to be associated with a wide array of endocrine and metabolic derangements more appropriately described as a syndrome, the polycystic ovarian syndrome (PCOS). The pathophysiology of PCOS lies in defective pulsatile secretion of hypothalamus GnRH, with a resultant predominant pituitary secretion of LH in relation to FSH. The elevated LH level stimulates an increased androgen synthesis in the theca cells. On the other hand, the low FSH level leads to (1) low aromatase activity in the granulosa cells where androgen is converted into estrogen, and (2) poor follicular development, increased follicular atresia and failure of ovulation. There is an increased peripheral tissue insulin resistance, hyperinsulinism, increased adiponectin hormone secretion by adipocytes, and dyslipidemia.

The diagnosis of PCOS is based on fulfillment of at least two of the following three criteria: (1) oligo-ovulation or anovulation manifested as oligomenorrhea or amenorrhea; (2) hyperandrogenism clinically (hirsutism) or hyperandrogenemia biochemically (raised free testosterone, and dehydroepiandrosterone-sulfate or DHEA-S); and (3) polycystic ovaries as defined on ultrasound scan where there are 12 or more follicles measuring 2–9 mm in diameter in at least one ovary or the total ovarian volume is greater than 10 cm^3.

Treatment of PCOS is based on the woman's desire of fertility. Combined estrogen-progestogen contraceptive pills are the treatment of choice for women not attempting for conception immediately. For those attempting for pregnancy immediately, treatment for ovulation induction can be achieved with clomiphene citrate or metformin. Lifestyle management with appropriate diet and physical exercise also plays an integral role in the overall treatment of PCOS. Surgical management with ovarian wedge resection or ovarian drilling is rarely indicated in women not responding adequately to medical treatment.

PCOS is associated with metabolic syndrome of hypertension, hyperglycemia and/or diabetes mellitus, hyperlipidemia and an increased risk of endometrial hyperplasia and adenocarcinoma. These women should be placed under long-term medical surveillance.

Illustration of Some Conditions that can Cause Oligo-menorrhea

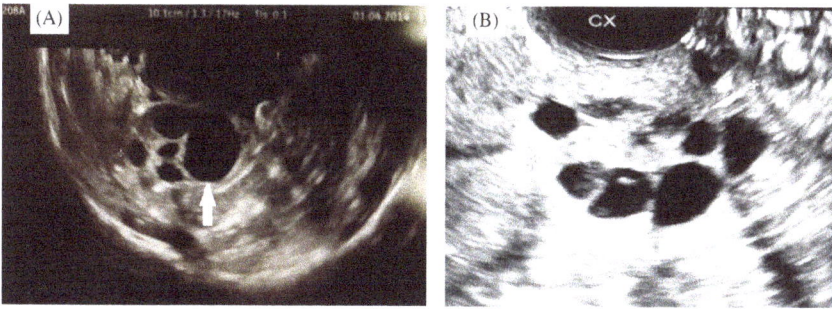

This panel of photographs of ultrasound scans shows a dominant follicle in a normal ovulatory ovary (marked by white arrow in panel (A), and multiple follicles located at the periphery of the ovary in PCOS in panel (B).

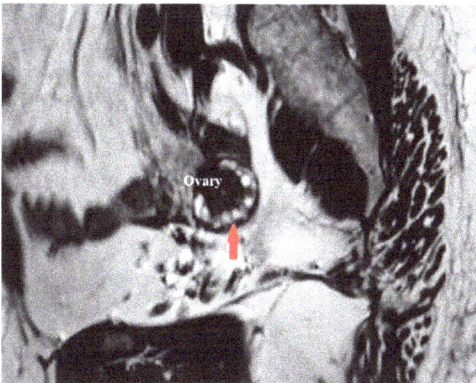

This photograph of a section of MR imaging shows the typical appearance of a polycystic ovary with multiple small follicles arranged at the periphery of the ovary (marked by red arrow). Note: This photograph was taken from a woman being investigated for other reasons as routine MR imaging for diagnosis of PCOS is not warranted.

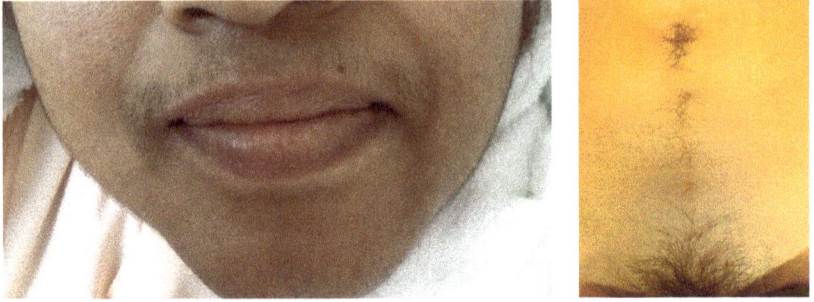

This panel of photographs shows the appearance of facial hirsutism and the male pattern of pubic hair distribution in a case of PCOS.

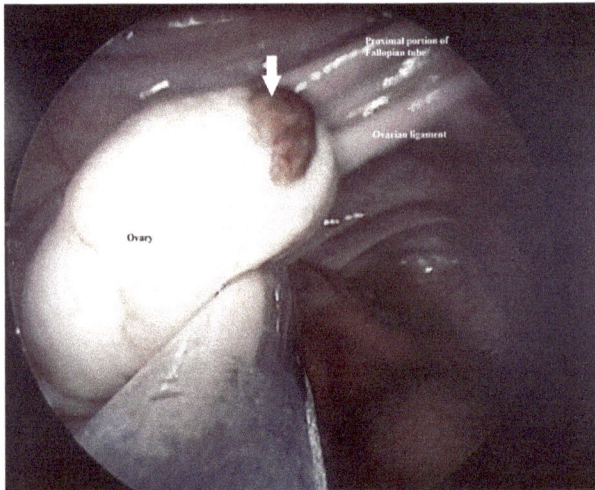

This photograph of a laparoscopy shows an ovary with a smooth capsule. The woman had a clinical diagnosis of PCOS and was treated with oral clomiphene citrate. The photograph shows evidence of ovulation as pointed out by the white arrow.

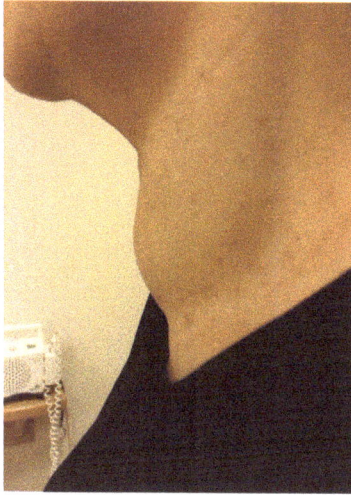

This photograph shows a woman with a goiter.

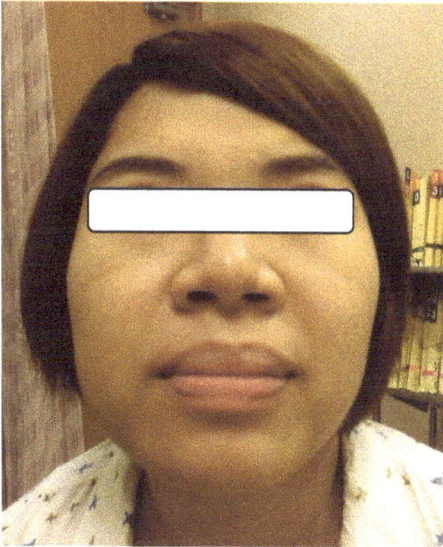

This photograph shows the coarse facial features in a 26-year-old woman with acromegaly and oligomenorrhea. Comparison of the features in photograph taken at different years is revealing of the changes in the features.

CASE 3 — SECONDARY AMENORRHEA

A 26-year-old woman complains of not experiencing a menstruation for nine months.

- What is the definition of secondary amenorrhea?
- What conditions may cause secondary amenorrhea?
- What are the initial investigations?

What is the Definition of Secondary Amenorrhea?

Secondary amenorrhea is defined as cessation of menstruation, not due to pregnancy, for either (i) a duration of six or more months following regular menstruation previously, or (ii) for a duration of 12 or more months following oligomenorrhea previously. The commonest causes of secondary amenorrhea are physiological conditions of pregnancy and lactation. Lactating women have infrequent and erratic ovulation. Amenorrhea may persist for as long as a woman remains lactating. Some women, after an average duration of six months of lactation, resume menstruation.

The prevalence of secondary amenorrhea as defined above is 3% overall, 3–5% among college students, 5–60% among endurance athletes, and 19–44% among ballet dancers.

What Conditions may Cause Secondary Amenorrhea?

Pathological conditions causing secondary amenorrhea can be grouped according to the anatomy sites of the lesion (common causes are marked by asterisk):

(i) **Genital Tract Lesions**
- Asherman syndrome
- Cervical stenosis
- Vaginal adhesions
- Uterine irradiation
- Progestin-impregnated intra-uterine device.

(ii) **Ovarian Lesions**
- Primary ovarian failure*
- Ovarian irradiation or systemic cytotoxic chemotherapy*.

(iii) **Pituitary Lesions**
- Prolactinoma*
- PCOS*
- Sheehan syndrome
- Autoimmune hypophysitis
- Pituitary radiation
- Panhypopituitarism
- Hypothyroidism*.

(iv) **Hypothalamic Lesions**

Organic causes:
- Craniopharyngioma or teratoma
- Cranial trauma

Functional causes:
- Eating disorders (Anorexia/bulimia)*
- Extreme obesity*
- Chronic disease
- Weight loss*
- Malnutrition

- Extreme physical exercise
- Severe stress*
- Depression*
- Psychotropic drug therapy
- Recreational drug abuse.

What are the Initial Investigations for this Condition?

Women with secondary amenorrhea should be investigated for the aim of management of the underlying medical conditions:

(i) **History**
- Menarche and previous menstrual history
- Eating and exercise patterns
- Changes in weight
- Chronic illness and medication use
- Presence of galactorrhea
- Symptoms of androgen excess, abnormal thyroid function, or vasomotor instability.

(ii) **Physical Examination**
- Measure patient's height, weight, and body mass index
- Thyroid examination
- Look out for signs of hyperandrogenism: acne and virilization (hirsutism, clitoromegaly)
- Genital tract outflow obstruction
- Hypoestrogenism: thin vaginal mucosa
- Dysmorphic features such as webbed neck or low hairline (Turner syndrome).

(iii) **Initial Investigation**
- Pregnancy test
- Serum luteinizing hormone, follicle-stimulating hormone, prolactin, and thyroid-stimulating hormone levels.
- For hyperandrogenic patients, serum-free and total testosterone and dehydroepiandrosterone sulfate (DHEAS)

- Patient with short stature: karyotype analysis
- Pelvic ultrasonography to identify structural abnormalities of reproductive tract organs.

Selected Diseases

1. Asherman Syndrome

Joseph Asherman first described, in 1948, a condition in a group of women who experienced cyclic pelvic pain with absence of menstruation. Asherman syndrome now refers to intrauterine adhesions during the reproductive life of a woman but excludes those in whom adhesions are intentionally induced for therapeutic purposes. In this condition, damage to basal layer of the endometrium is seen with replacement of stroma with fibrosis, and the glands are sparse and cystically dilated with cubo-columnar epithelium. The failure of development of the functional layer of the endometrium manifests in absence of menstruation.

The most common cause of Asherman syndrome is curettage on a pregnant uterus such as surgery for induced abortion, miscarriage or post-partum hemorrhage. The incidence following these procedures is estimated to range from 7% to 20%. The occurrence rate of Asherman syndrome following instrumentation of a non-pregnant uterus such as diagnostic curettage and myomectomy ranges from 0.2 to 1.6%. Rare infection of the uterus with tuberculosis and schistosomiasis is also known to be able to cause Asherman syndrome.

Depending on the extent of intrauterine adhesions, the clinical presentation includes secondary amenorrhea, oligomenorrhea, and subfertility. There is also associated cyclic pelvic pain.

Investigations will show a normal range of serum estrogen, FSH and LH levels appropriate for the time of menstrual phase. Pelvic ultrasound scan and magnetic resonance imaging technique may demonstrate the presence of intrauterine adhesions but the definitive diagnosis is confirmed on hysteroscopy.

The treatment of Asherman syndrome is surgical excision of the adhesions followed by insertion of an intrauterine contraceptive device to prevent post-surgical occlusion of the cavity. The development of a functional layer is further enhanced with estrogen therapy. Returning of menstruation depends on the extent of remaining endometrial basalis but the prognosis for pregnancy is poor.

2. Premature Ovarian Failure

Ovarian hypogonadism or primary ovarian insufficiency is also commonly known as premature ovarian failure. It is defined as loss of ovarian function between the age of menarche and 40 years old, although occasional menstruation and spontaneous pregnancy may be seen. This is distinguishable from premature menopause in which cessation of menstruation and loss of capacity of spontaneous pregnancy are permanent.

The most common causes of primary ovarian failure are idiopathic (46%), Turner syndrome (30%), type-2 autoimmune polyendocrinopathy (8%), and familiar (6%).

Premature ovarian failure manifests symptoms of estrogen deficiency and health problems of osteoporosis and cardiovascular disorders. Diagnosis is based on elevated serum levels of FSH and LH and a low circulating level of estradiol, and histological examination of the ovary revealing absence of primordial follicles. Further investigation with karyotyping may be warranted in some patients.

Premature ovarian failure is treated with estrogen-progestogen replacement. Child bearing can be achieved through ovum or embryo donation programs.

3. Functional Hypothalamus Amenorrhea (FHA)

FHA is the most common cause of secondary amenorrhea and is responsible for 35% of reversible secondary amenorrhea. It is characterized hormonally by low estrogen and androstenedione levels, increased FSH/LH ratio and suppressed LH pulsatile frequency and amplitude. The gonadotrophin deficiency is functional and partial as demonstrated by response to GnRH agonist test. It is a consequence of low dietary intake (anorexia nervosa, prolonged mild fat intake restriction), intensive physical exercise, weight loss, and mental or psychological stresses. The role of diet in FHA is likely to be mediated via several neuroendocrine factors, most notably neuropeptide Y, leptin and ghrelin. Neuropeptide Y is produced, predominantly, by the arcuate and paraventricular nuclei of the hypothalamus. It controls the body energy balance and has a direct regulatory effect on GnRH release. The level of neuropeptide Y is low in FHA women. Leptin, a peptide secreted by adipocytes, has a stimulatory role on the GnRH pulsatility and a stimulatory effect on pituitary gonadotrope cells. Its secretion is increased in obesity and decreased in starvation. The circulating leptin level is lower in women with FHA compared to women matched with age, BMI and body fat composition. Ghrelin is an acylated peptide secreted by oxyntic cells of the stomach and duodenum and in the hypothalamus and pituitary gland. Ghrelin stimulates appetite, reduces fat utilization and inhibits pulsatile secretion of LH. In women with FHA, raised ghrelin level is stimulated by inadequate feeding pattern and negative energy balance.

On the other hand, intensive physical exercises, weight loss and mental stresses increase endogenous ß-endorphin release in the central nervous system. ß-endorphin inhibits pulsatile GnRH and LH release.

4. Hyperprolactinemia

Prolactin is a hormone produced by lactotroph cells of the pituitary gland. The physiological regulation of prolactin secretion is via the hypothalamic dopamine inhibitory pathway. Hyperprolactinemia is a condition of persistent elevation of serum prolactin level after excluding pregnancy and lactation. In women, the most common presentation of hyperprolactinemia is oligomenorrhea, secondary amenorrhea, galactorrhea, or infertility. Manifestation of mass effects from pressure of enlarged pituitary adenoma on optic chiasma with visual field defects is uncommon but important for clinical management. There may be features of chronic hypogonadism: loss of libido, habitual abortion and hypoetrogenic osteopenia.

Pathological causes of chronic hyperprolactinemia include:

- Pituitary adenoma — most commonly microadenoma
- Primary hypothyroidism — 40% of patients with primary hypothyroidism are hyperprolactinemic
- Chronic renal failure — 30% of women with renal failure and 80% of women on renal dialysis are hyperprolactinemic.
- Dopamine receptor inhibitory drugs — phenothiazines, butyrophenones, metoclopramide
- Hypothalamic-pituitary axis disorders — craniopharyngiomas, and gliomas; mental/emotional stresses.

Hyperprolactinemia is diagnosed on elevated serum prolactin level on two or more occasions. An underlying cause of hyperprolactinemia must be determined with a detailed clinical history and drug history, physical examination, and appropriate laboratory investigations. In the absence of an identifiable cause of hyperprolactinemia, MR imaging studies will provide an excellent evaluation of pituitary sellar disorder and hypothalamic lesions.

The first principle in treatment of hyperprolactinemia remains the correction of its underlying causes. In other cases, asymptomatic hyperprolactinemia may be managed expectantly. Pituitary microadenoma with mild hyperprolactinemia rarely progresses to macroadenomas, regardless of age of presentation. In the absence of a microadenoma, less than 20% of women with mild hyperprolactinaemia showed a doubling of serum prolactin level on long-term follow up.

Women with amenorrhea, infertility and feature of hypogonadism should be treated with dopamine agonist, bromocryptin or cabergolin. Bromocryptine is effective in 90% of cases, with normalization of serum prolactin level and reduction in the size of adenoma. In women with no desire for pregnancy, combined estrogen-progestogen contraceptives or estrogen replacement therapy for management of hypoganodism is an alternative treatment of hyperprolactinemia.

Illustration of Some Conditions that can Cause Secondary Amenorrhea

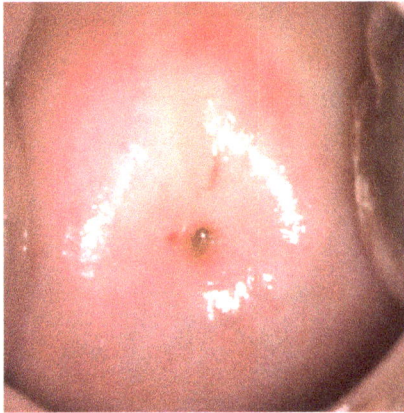

This 32-year-old woman had a cervical intraepithelial neoplasia grade 3 involving the endocervical canal. After a CO_2 laser cone biopsy of the cervix, her menstruation gradually diminished in quantity and, 4 months later, stopped completely. This was associated with a history of worsening cyclic dysmenorrhea-like lower abdominal cramps. This colpo-photograph shows severe stenosis of the external os of the cervix. The stenosis involved a complete obliteration of the lower portion of the endocervical canal (not shown on this picture) which obstructed the outflow of menstrual blood, a condition known as secondary cryptomenorrhea.

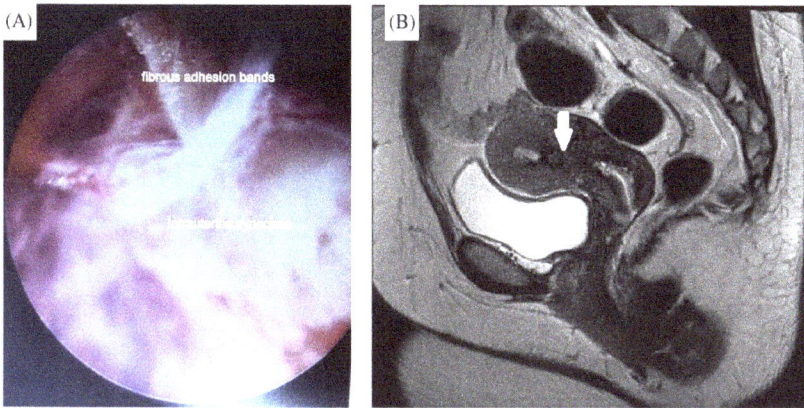

This 39-year-old woman had an evacuation of the uterus for a first trimester miscarriage. She failed to resume menstruation in the following 6 months. Her pelvic organs were normal on clinical examination and serum level of FSH, LH estrogen, prolactin, TSH and free T4 were normal. A clinical diagnosis of Asherman syndrome was made. Photograph panel (A) demonstrates intrauterine adhesions during a hysterosopy. Panel (B) shows obliteration of the endometrial cavity by adhesions on a T-2 weighted MR image (marked by white arrow).

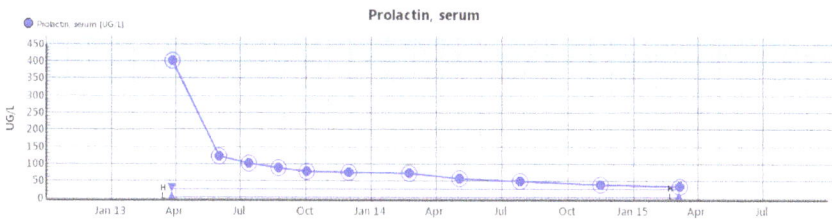

This chart documented the change in serum prolactin levels during the 12-month period of treatment with bromocryptin. The patient resumed normal menstruation within 3 months of initiation of the treatment.

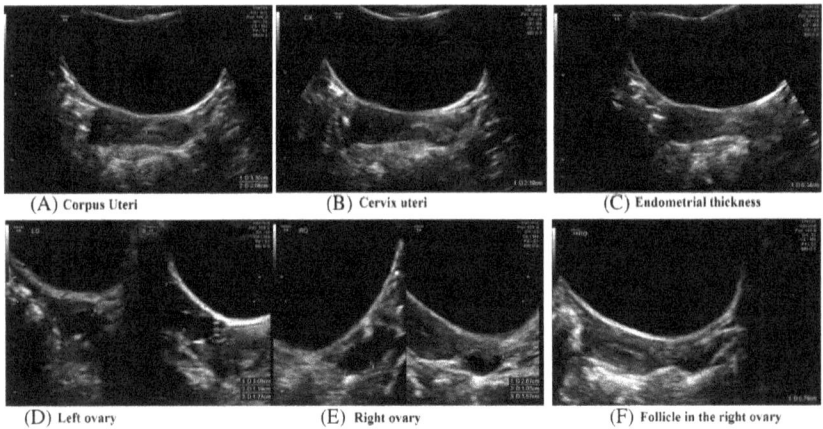

(A) Corpus Uteri   (B) Cervix uteri   (C) Endometrial thickness

(D) Left ovary   (E) Right ovary   (F) Follicle in the right ovary

This 22-year-old woman was amenorrheic for 18 months. She was a well and fit woman who performed aerobic exercises and 5-km jogging more than 5 times a week. She measured 1.56 m in height and 45.7 kg in weight. The calculated BMI was 18.8.

This panel of photographs of a transabdominal ultrasound scan shows that the volume of the uterus was small (14.5 mL), endometrial thickness was low (3.4 mm), and the ovaries contained multiple small follicles (3–9 mm in diameters).

Her endocrinology profile was normal:

FSH = 6.1 U/L (follicular phase 1.0–14.0 U/L0

LH = 1.2 U/L (follicular phase 1.0–7.5 U/L)

Estradiol = 78.3 pmol/L (follicular phase 46–607 pmol/L)

Prolactin = 8.9 μg/L (normal range 5.0–27.7 μg/L)

TSH = 3.56 MU/L (normal range 0.65–3.70 MU/L0

Free T4 = 10.1 pmol/L (normal range 8.8–14.4 pmol/L)

Her condition was diagnosed as functional hypothalamic amenorrhea (FHA).

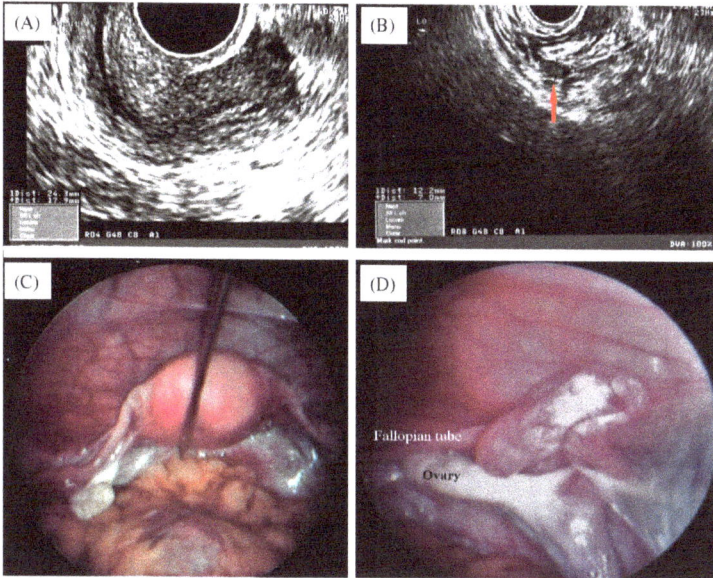

An 18-year-old girl gave a history of several menstruations during the first year since menarche at the age of 13 years. There was no further menstruation for the ensuing four years. There was no other relevant medical, surgical or psychiatric history. Physical examination showed a well and fit woman with no dysmorphic features. The secondary sexual characteristics were normal. The photograph (panel (A)) shows the uterus measured 24 mm in longitudinal section, 18 mm in antero-posterior distance, and 27 mm in the transverse diameter, or a computed volume of 6.07 cm^3. The endometrial thickness was 2.7 mm. The right ovary was not visible. The left ovary measured 12 mm in length, 7 mm in antero-posterior distance and 9 mm in transverse diameter, or 0.39 cm^3 in volume (panel (B), red arrow). The anatomy of the pelvis on laparoscopy was shown in panels (C) (uterus and left ovary) and (D) (right ovary and fallopian tube). Serum biochemistry profile and investigations showed:

Hormone	Result	Normal Range
FSH	26	3–20 mIU/mL (follicular phase)
LH	20	2–15 mIU/mL (follicular phase)
Estradiol	8	9–221 pg/mL (follicular phase)
Progesterone	0.3	0.1–1.5 ng/mL (follicular phase)
Free testosterone	0.2	0.07–13.5 pmol/L
DHEA-SO4	2.7	0.9–11.2 umol/L
Prolactin	21	0.5–18.1 ng/mL
Thyroid stimulation hormone	0.9	0.45–6.20 mIU/mL
Chromosome karyotyping	46 XY, no deletions of translocation detected.	
Right and left ovarian biopsy	Absence of primordial follicles.	

This woman had secondary amenorrhea from premature ovarian insufficiency probably as a consequence of viral oophoritis or autoimmune disorders.

CASE 4 — INTERMENSTRUAL BLEEDING

A 30-year-old woman complains of vaginal bleeding in between menstruations.

- Is intermenstrual bleeding normal?
- What are the common causes of intermenstrual bleeding?
- How should her symptoms be investigated?

Is Intermenstrual Bleeding (IMB) Normal?

During the reproductive life-span, almost every woman will experience some changes in the pattern of menstrual flow and menstrual cycle. In the absence of a pregnancy or therapeutic hormonal influence, any uterine bleeding that occurs between otherwise a normal pattern of menstruation is referred to as intermenstrual bleeding.

Two types of IMB can be observed: the bleeding that occurs once only in between otherwise normal menstruations, and those that occurs on and off in between menstruations. The former type of IMB is physiological and occurs in approximately 20–30% of women or 1–2% of all menstrual cycles. Typically, it occurs between day-10 and day-16 of the menstrual cycle and lasts for 12–72 hours. The bleeding is usually scanty or light. It is often described as spotting of blood.

Physiological IMB is associated with ovulation. There is a surge in serum level of estrogen towards the end of the follicular phase. The negative feedback of estrogen to the pituitary gland and the associated surge in luteinizing hormone cause an abrupt dip in the circulating estrogen level just before ovulation. This change in circulating estrogen level precipitates breaking down of endometrium with a resultant uterine bleeding.

What are the Common Causes of Intermenstrual Bleeding?

Irregular intermenstrual bleeding which occurs without a recognized pattern between normal menstruations are not associated with ovulation and maybe caused by a wide range of pathology:

(i) **Ovarian Disorders**
   • Anovulation

(ii) **Uterine Disorders**
   • Endometrial polyp
   • Fibroids
   • Endometrial cancer
   • Sarcoma.

(iii) **Endocrine Disorder**
   • Thyroid disorders

(iv) **Infection**
   • Endometritis

(v) **Iatrogenic**
   • Contraceptive pills
   • Intrauterine contraceptive device
   • Anticoagulation.

(vi) **Other Non-uterine Causes of Abnormal Vaginal Bleeding**
   • Cervical polyp
   • Cervical endometriosis
   • Cervical cancer
   • Vaginal tumor
   • Vulvar tumor
   • Genital warts.

How should her Symptoms be Investigated?

(i) **History**
- Presence or absence of recognizable regular menstruation pattern
- Detailed history of bleeding pattern in relation to the menstrual cycle
- Provocative factors for the bleeding, such as sexual intercourse
- Associated symptoms, in particular pelvic pain, dyspareunia
- Use of medications, including female sex hormones, anticoagulants
- History of cervical screening.

(ii) **Physical Examination**
- Thyroid examination
- Presence or absence of abdominal-pelvic masses
- Presence or absence of lower genital tract lesions
- Uterine size and contour
- Adnexal and pelvic tenderness, nodularity or masses.

(iii) **Laboratory Investigations: Initial Investigation should include the following:**
- Cervical screening, if not done within the previous one year
- Swabs from vagina and endocervical canal for bacteriological investigations if cervicitis or endometritis is clinically evident
- Pelvic ultrasound scan for uterine lesions and other pelvic abnormalities.

Selected Conditions

1. Anovulatory Bleeding. Irregular intermenstrual bleeding maybe a manifestation of anovulation. In the early years of menstrual life, anovulation is associated with inadequate function of the hypothalamic-pituitary-ovarian axis. At the other extreme, or the perimenopausal period, anovulation reflects the gradual failing of the ovaries. In between the two extremes of reproductive life, the commonest cause of anovulation is polycystic ovarian syndrome, which presents more frequently as oligomenorrhea and secondary amenorrhea than intermenstrual bleeding.

Normal menstruation is the result of necrosis and shedding of the entire luteinized functional layer of the endometrium as a result of progesterone withdrawal, whereas the anovulatory cycle gives rise to a state of prolonged unopposed estrogenic stimulation of endometrium. The irregular patchy necrosis and shedding of superficial layer of the proliferative endometrium result in IMB.

2. Endometrial Polyps. These are pedunculated or sessile endo-metrial overgrowth consisting of endometrium, stroma and blood vessels. They can occur singly or in multiple numbers and the dimension ranges from several millimeters to a few centimeters. They are rarely malignant except in the high-risk population where up to 10% of the polyps may be malignant. The etiology of endo-metrial polyp is unknown but the prevalence seems to increase with age during the reproductive life. Depending on the study populations, the prevalence of endometrial polyps ranges from 7% to 30%. Other risk factors include infertility, hypertension, obesity and consumption of tamoxifen. Use of contraceptive pills contain-ing a progestogen with high anti-estrogenic property seems to confer some protective effect against endometrial polyps.

Most endometrial polyps are asymptomatic. In others, the most common manifestation of the polyps is abnormal uterine bleeding, including post-menopausal bleeding.

Transvaginal ultrasound scan remains the most informative clini-cal investigation with a sensitivity of 100%, specificity of 70% and negative predictive value of 100%. Hysteroscopy directed biopsy and histopathology evaluation are the most reliable diagnostic procedures.

Asymptomatic endometrial polyps of less than 10 mm in dimension carry a high rate of spontaneous regression. They can be managed expectantly. Symptomatic or large endometrial polyps can be removed by hysteroscopic polypectomy, hysteroscopic polyp resection, or rarely, in the presence of other prevailing indi-cation, by a hysterectomy.

Illustration of Some Conditions that can Cause IMB

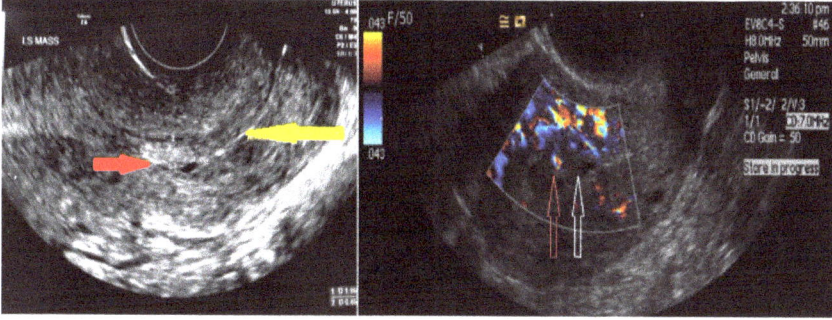

This panel of photographs of transvaginal ultrasound scans shows an endometrial polyp (panel on the left side). The photographs in the panel on the right is the color Doppler scan which shows the blood flow (red arrow) within the polyp (white arrow).

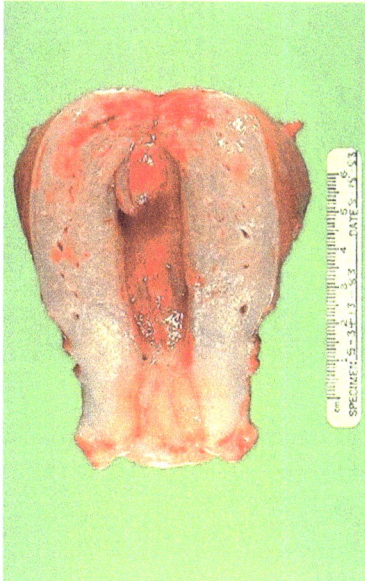

This photograph of a hysterectomy specimen shows an endometrial polyp at the fundus region of the uterine cavity.

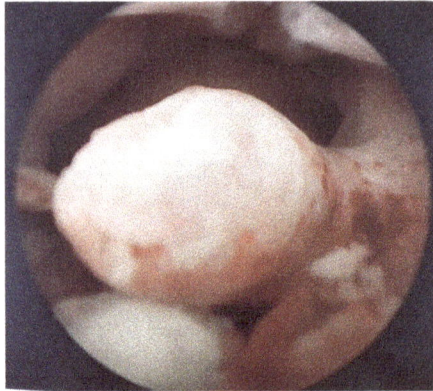

This photograph of a hysteroscopy shows the appearance of a pedunculated endometrial polyp at the fundus region of the uterine cavity. It was a fibroid polyp.

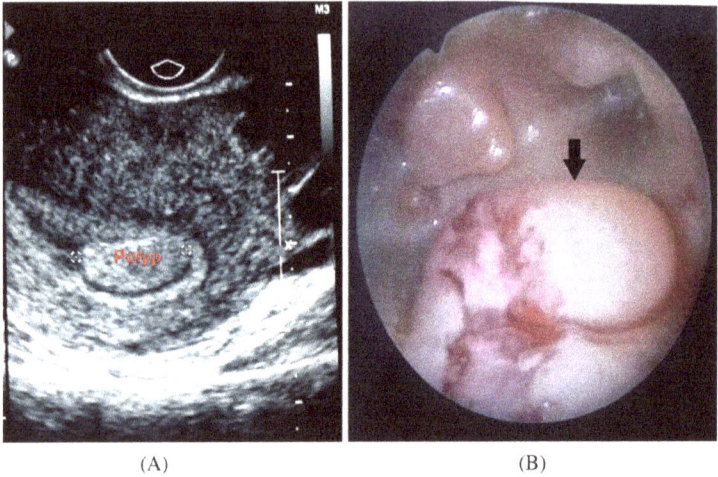

(A)   (B)

This panel of photographs shows (panel (A)) a uterine polyp, which was confirmed (marked by black arrow) on hysteroscopy in panel (B).

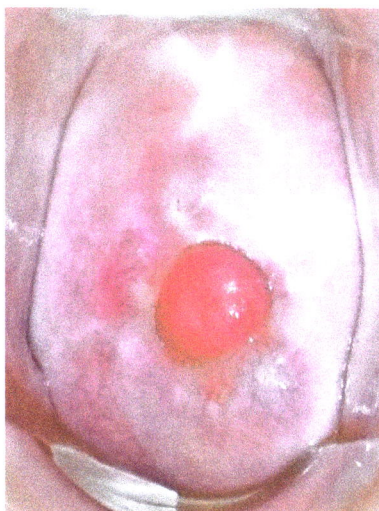

This photograph shows a cervical polyp which presented with irregular spotting of blood per vaginum.

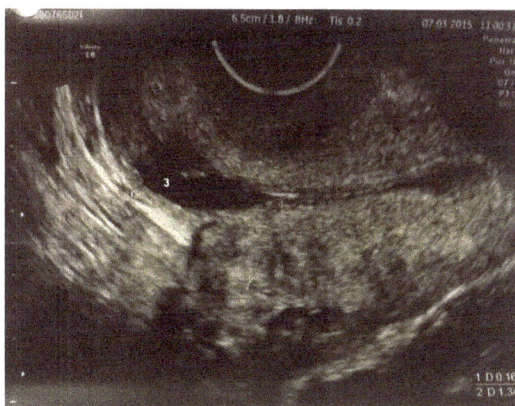

A photograph of a transvaginal ultrasound scan of the uterus showing a LSCS scar defect with a thin anterior uterine wall (marked "1"), compared to the normal myometrial thickness (marked "2"). A collection of fluid at the defect measured 1.9 cm × 0.6 cm × 1.8 cm was also demonstrated (marked "3").

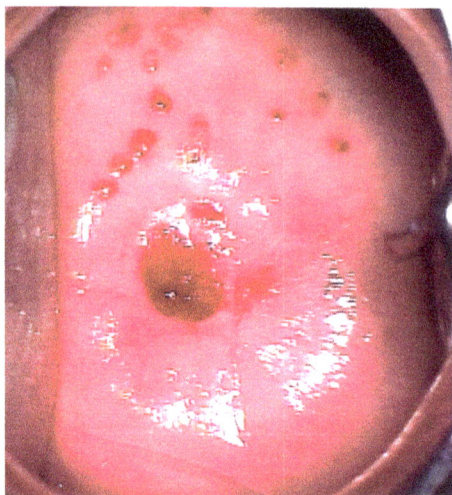

This woman complained of irregular spotting of blood per vaginum. The symptoms were most prominent for one week before and one week after menstruation. The photograph shows multiple endometriotic spots on the ectocervix.

CASE 5 — IRREGULAR MENSTRUATIONS

A 45-year-old married woman with two children complains of irregular menstruations for the past three months.

- What specific menstrual history would be informative?
- What conditions may explain her symptom?

What Specific Menstrual History would be Informative?

Irregular menstruation is one of the most imprecise symptoms in gynecology. An examination of the patient's menstrual calendar is the only way to establish the symptom correctly.

It is important to establish if there is a recognizable menstrual flow with normal characteristics in term of the quantity, quality and duration of blood loss. The cycle length can be determined by calculating the interval duration between the dates of onset of each bleeding. This allows irregular bleeding to be classified into one of the following patterns:

  (i) Cyclic bleeding with variable cycle intervals
 (ii) Menstrual cycle interrupted by intermenstrual bleeding
(iii) Menstruation complicated by premenstrual bleeding
 (iv) Menstruation associated with postmenstrual bleeding
  (v) Erratic bleeding with no cyclic pattern
 (vi) Post-coital bleeding, and
(vii) Post-menopausal bleeding.

What Conditions may Explain her Symptom?

Conditions causing irregular menstruation could be physiological or pathological. The average length of a menstrual cycle is 28 days, comprising 14 days of follicular development and 14 days of luteal function. The duration of physiological function of corpus luteum shows a small range of variation. In contrast, the follicular phase shows wide variations, ranging from 7 days to 21 days. Consequently, the physiological range of menstrual cycle length varies from 21 days to 35 days. For an individual woman, this variation manifests as irregular pattern of menstruation on calendar dates but a cyclic pattern is recognizable on close scrutiny of menstrual calendar.

On the other hand, a non-cyclic bleeding or erratically irregular menstruation is an ominous sign of significant pathology. It warrants a thorough clinical evaluation to reach an accurate diagnosis.

The causes of abnormal uterine bleeding are classified by FIGO and summarized in the acronym of "PALM-COEIN" to include Polyp, Adenomyosis, Leiomyoma, Malignancy and hyperplasia, Coagulopathy, Ovulatory dysfunction, Endometrial, Iatrogenic, and Not-yet-classified.

Among women referred to gynecologists for abnormal perimenopausal bleeding, the pathologic diagnosis included disordered proliferative endometrium (20%), secretory endometrium (15%), simple endometrial hyperplasia without atypia (30%), complex hyperplasia with atypia (5%), endometritis (15%), polyps (10%) and cancer in some instances. Features that may be suggestive of abnormal perimenopausal bleeding include excessively heavy and prolonged bleeding, increasing dysmenorrhea, intermenstrual bleeding and post-coital bleeding.

(i) Anovulation of Menopausal Transition: ovarian follicle atresia occurs throughout a woman's reproductive years. The diminished follicle reserve after 40 years old may present with poor ovarian response to pituitary FSH stimulation and an increased frequency of anovulatory cycles. This state of transition to menopause is commonly referred to as perimenopause. Characteristically, the menstrual pattern initially changes to shorter cycles for a varying period of time before the cycles become prolonged. The final menstruation marks the onset of menopause. During perimenopause, there is a marked variation in quantity of menstrual flow and, frequently, associated with premenstrual spotting of blood. These changes are physiological but clinicians must be alerted to differential diagnosis of abnormal uterine bleeding.

(ii) PCOS: irregular menstruation is one of the most common manifestations of PCOS. It is estimated that 20% of PCOS women show amenorrhea and many others show oligomenorrhea. However, irregular menstruation may occur as the unopposed estrogenic stimulation leads to thickened endometrium which readily undergoes superficial sloughing and shedding. In long-standing cases, there may be endometrial hyperplasia. PCOS is one of the most common causes of endometrial adenocarcinoma in women below 40 years old.

(iii) Early Pregnancy Complications: the incidence of pregnancy failure increases with the age of women and up to 40% of pregnancies in women above 40 years old end in miscarriages. Also, 1% of pregnancies are extrauterine or ectopic in location. Early pregnancy failure often does not show a period of amenorrhea and the woman maybe unaware of the pregnancy except an erratic uterine bleeding. A high index of suspicion for the diagnosis is needed when a woman complains of erratic uterine bleeding in a recent onset. The diagnosis can be confirmed on a urinary pregnancy test or serum β-HCG determination and ultrasound scan of the uterus and pelvic organs.

(iv) Endometrial Hyperplasia: endometrial hyperplasia arises from a state of estrogen stimulation unopposed by progesterone. There is excess endometrial glandular proliferation in relation to the stroma. Based on histological architectural complexity and cellular abnormality, endometrial hyperplasia is further classified into simple hyperplasia, simple hyperplasia with atypia, complex hyperplasia, and complex hyperplasia with atypia. In 2014, the new FIGO classification simplified these conditions into two categories: benign endometrial hyperplasia which encompasses the previously known simple hyperplasia without atypia and complex hyperplasia without atypia; and atypical endometrial hyperplasia which encompasses simple hyperplasia and complex hyperplasia with atypia. These states represent the spectrum of endometrial pathology before development of endometrioid adenocarcinoma of the endometrium. In untreated state, the rate of progression to adenocarcinoma is 1% for simple hyperplasia, 3% for complex hyperplasia, 8% for simple hyperplasia with atypia, and 25% for complex hyperplasia with atypia. In some reports, co-existing well-differentiated endometrioid adeno-carcinoma is found in 20% to 40% of complex hyperplasia with atypia.

Endometrial hyperplasia can present with erratic menstruation or heavy menstrual bleeding in pre-menopausal women, or with post-menopausal bleeding. Ultrasound scan may detect the thickened endometrium but the diagnosis is based on histology. Several devices are available for endometrial sampling or biopsy in the office and they are preferred to formal dilatation and curettage.

(v) Other Causes of Erratic Menstruation
- Progestin
- IUD
- Anticoagulation
- Thyroid disorders
- Hyperprolactinemia

Illustration of Some Conditions that can Cause Irregular Menstruations

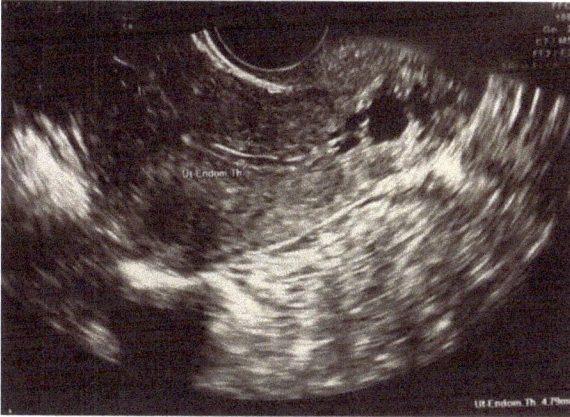

Irregular menstruation reflects a potential pathology in the endometrium. Anatomy of endometrium is well demonstrable on ultrasound scan. This photograph of a transvaginal ultrasound scan of the uterus illustrates the measurement of the endometrial thickness.

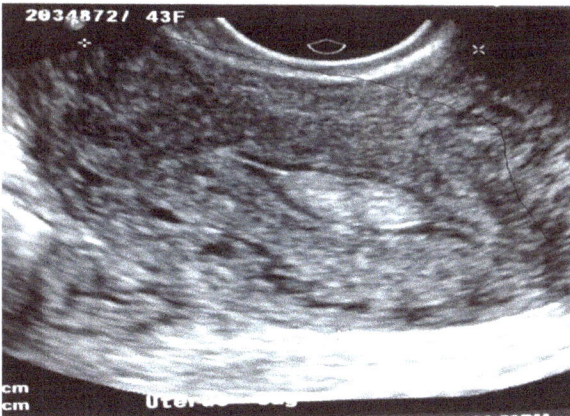

This photograph of an ultrasound scan shows an endometrial polyp in a 43-year-old woman complaining of erratic uterine bleeding.

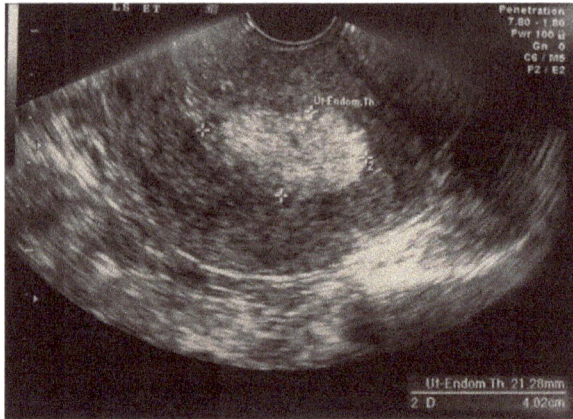

This photograph of a transvaginal ultrasound scan of the uterus in a case of a 45-year-old woman complaining of irregular menstruation, shows a markedly thickened endometrium of 21.2 mm. Histological diagnosis was mandatory. It showed an endometrial cancer.

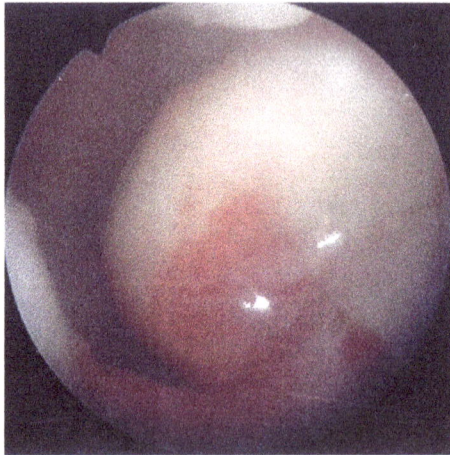

This photograph of hysteroscopy shows a submucous fibroid extending into intrauterine cavity as the cause of irregular menstruation in this woman.

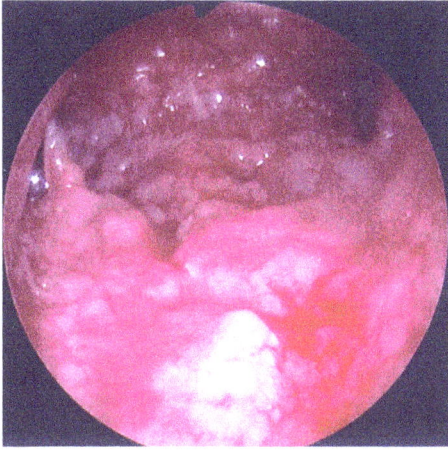

A photograph of hystoscopic examination shows the irregular and markedly thickened endometrium from a case of simple endometrial hyperplasia.

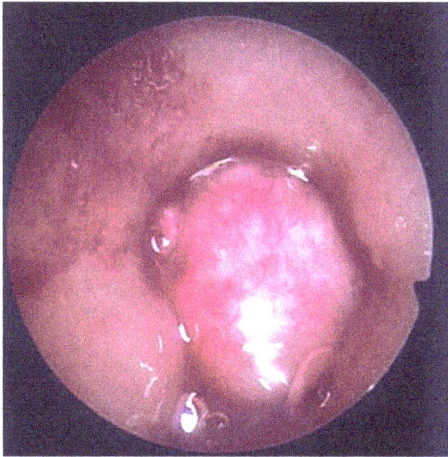

A photograph of hystoscopy shows a large endometrial polyp with prominent vascular surface appearance. Pathological examination confirmed that it was an endometrioid adenocarcinoma.

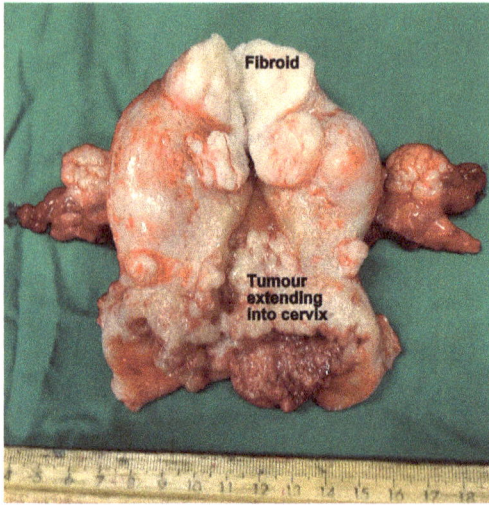

This photograph from THBSO specimen shows a large endometrial carcinoma involving the cervix (stage-II). The photograph also shows the presence of several intramural fibroids which can confuse the diagnosis of her erratic menstruation.

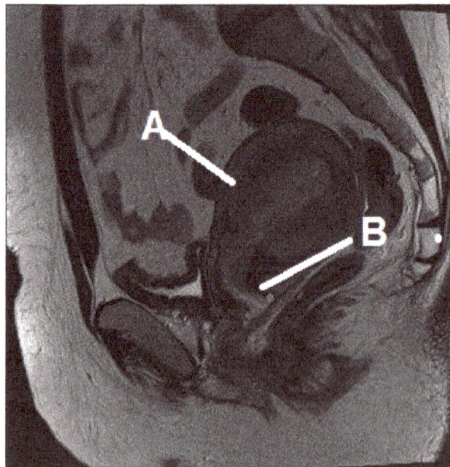

A MRI-T2 image showing an endometrial carcinoma in the fundal region of the uterine cavity. The tumor was confined to the endometrium.

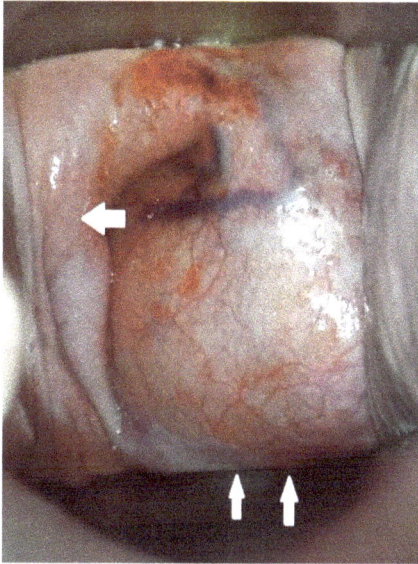

This 35-year-old woman complained of prolonged scanty vaginal bleeding following a normal onset menstruation. A speculum examination revealed a large Nabothian cyst (marked with two small arrows). The surface epithelium was inflammed with abundant fine capillaries and engorged superficial veins. Evidence of scanty bleeding was seen in this photograph. The cervix on the right hand side (marked with a thick white arrow) was normal in appearance.

CASE 6 — HEAVY MENSTRUAL BLEEDING

A 40-year-old para-1 woman complains of heavy menstruation for six months.

- What physiological mechanisms control the normal menstruation?
- How much blood loss is considered heavy menstrual bleeding?
- What conditions may explain this patient's complaint?
- Outline the management of idiopathic HMB.

What Physiological Mechanisms Control the Normal Menstruation?

Menstruation is uterine bleeding from shedding of the endometrium and is subject to physiological control as seen in any wound bleeding: hemostasis, vasoconstriction and tissue repair.

Hemostasis. The first step in controlling bleeding from breakdown of spiral arterioles in the sloughing endometrium is activation of platelet aggregation and formation of platelet plugs to temporarily seal off the vessels. This is followed by activation of the cascade of clotting factors and formation of fibrin. These processes, however, start less rapidly in the endometrium compared to wounds seen elsewhere. On the other hand, the fibrinolytic process mediated via plasminogen activation by the urokinase-type (uPA) and tissue-type plasminogen (tPA) activators starts rapidly to prevent formation of clots which may otherwise obliterate the endometrial cavity. tPA level is higher in the endometrium than other tissues and its activity is inhibited by progesterone.

Vasoconstriction. In the first 20 hours of menstruation, bleeding is controlled by intense constriction of the damaged spiral arterioles.

49

Prostaglandin F2α (PG F2α) constricts while prostaglandin E_2 (PGE$_2$) dilates the blood vessels. Damaged endometrium releases endothelin which, by inducing contraction of vascular and myometrial smooth muscles, also plays an important part in maintaining vasoconstriction. PG F2α enhances endometrial release of endothelin.

Endometrial Repair. Endometrial regeneration starts on day-2 and completes the re-epithelialization of the endometrium by day-5 of menstruation. Two processes play an important role in endometrial regeneration: (1) estrogen-dependent endometrial and stromal proliferation; and (2) tissue hypoxia induced endometrial angiogenic growth factors, predominantly the vascular endothelium growth factor (VEGF) and fibroblast growth factors (FGF).

How Much Blood Loss is Considered Heavy Menstrual Bleeding?

In a typical menstruation lasting three to eight days, there is an average total blood loss of 40 mL (range 37–43 mL). The majority of blood loss occurs within the first 48 hours of menstruation. Although both the cycle length and total amount of blood loss show a marked variation between women, they remain relatively constant for each individual, in particular for women between 20- and 40-years old.

Menstrual blood loss in excess of 80 mL leads to worsened quality of life of the woman from social inconvenience, work place absenteeism, and consequences of anemia. The condition is termed heavy menstrual bleeding (HMB) in preference to menorrhagia.

Approximately 9–14% of menstruating women ever experience HMB. The annual rate is at the lowest at 0.67% for the 12–24 year-olds and the highest at 5.4% for the 45–49 year-olds. The rate seems to be rising from the 25 year-olds to the 49 year-olds, probably by the rising incidence of uterine pathology with age.

The diagnosis of HMB is hinged on a patient's report of a change in the menstruation and the impact of the menstruation on her physical health and quality of life. The presence of HMB is supported by a reduced blood hemoglobin level. Quantification of menstrual blood loss is feasible only on research settings. Pictorial aids, useful clinical tools for monitoring progress of treatment, do not correlate with the actual amount of blood loss and do not provide a reliable semi-quantitative assessment of HMB.

What Conditions may Explain this Patient's Complaint?

The causes of HMB can be categorized on pathophysiological basis into dysfunctional uterine bleeding (DUB), pelvic pathology, medical disorders and coagulopathy:

Cause	Pathology
Idiopathic HMB	None apparent
Pelvic diseases	Uterine fibroids Uterine adenomyosis Endometrial polyps Intrauterine contraceptive device
Medical disorders	Hypothyroidism Cushing' disease Viral associated thrombocytopenia e.g. Dengue fever
Coagulopathy	Thrombocytopenic purpura Von Willebrand's disease Congenital clotting factor deficiency Iatrogenic: anti-coagulation therapy

Idiopathic Heavy Menstrual Bleeding. This is a preferred terminology for dysfunctional uterine bleeding (DUB). It is the commonest clinical presentation of HMB, in particular at the two extreme ends of the reproductive life. A woman is said to have idiopathic HMB if she is distressed physically or socio-economically by heavy menstrual blood loss without an organic cause or pregnancy.

It is estimated that 20% of idiopathic HMB involves anovulatory cycles. The menstrual cycle is irregular and HMB is painless. The pathophysiology is related to the lack of progesterone and persistent endometrial proliferation under the estrogenic influence. The increased endometrial thickness or hyperplasia and the absence of progesterone-induced PG F2α result in idiopathic HMB. In contrast, ovulatory idiopathic HMB is cyclic and may be painful. The pathophysiology is not well defined but is believed to be due to dysregulation of vasoconstriction. There is a demonstrable shift from endometrial secretion of vasoconstrictor PGF2α to vasodilator PGE_2 (increased PGE_2/PG F2α ratio), and a diminished endothelin level in the endometrium.

The diagnosis of idiopathic HMB is established on excluding HMB caused by medical conditions and pelvic diseases. Suspicion of uterine pathology should be raised in the presence of a clinical history of menstrual irregularity, intermenstrual bleeding, postcoital bleeding, pelvic pain or premenstrual pain, dyspareunia, and therapy with unopposed estrogen or tamoxifen. A carefully conducted physical examination is mandatory as it may reveal evidence of anemia, hypothyroidism, coagulopathy or pathology in the pelvis such as endometriosis, adenomyosis, pelvic inflammatory disease, uterine fibroids, cervical polyps or carcinoma of the cervix. The existence of pathology in the endometrial cavity can be detected by pelvic ultrasound scan, endometrial tissue assessment, and hysteroscopy.

A transvaginal ultrasound scan has a sensitivity of 96% and specificity of 89% of detecting a uterine and pelvic lesion. Magnetic resonance (MR) imaging, if performed, may also demonstrate uterine pathologies. Specific diagnosis of endometrial pathology, malignancy in particular, requires an endometrial biopsy. A number of endometrial samplers are available for this purpose in the office setting, such as Pipelle and endometrial explorer. These blind sampling techniques share a similar sensitivity as dilatation and curettage (D & C) procedure for diagnosis of endometrial carcinoma. Hystersocopic endometrial biopsy is superior to blind sampling for diagnosis of benign pathology such as submucous fibroids and polyps as the cause of HMB. Hysteroscopy is always accompanied with biopsy of the endometrium to exclude endometrial pathology. It is an operative procedure which also allows therapeutic procedure such as endometrial ablation or resection of a submucous fibroid to be performed.

Outline the Management of Idiopathic HMB

HMB accounts for 20% of gynecological consultations. Management of HMB can be divided into; (i) treatment of acute bleeding, and (ii) long-term therapy.

(i) **Acute Management.** Treatment of acute bleeding from idiopathic HMB includes prostaglandin synthetase inhibitors, anti-fibrinolytics and progestogen. The non-hormonal therapy is attractive to women as the treatment restricted to the menstrual phase is devoid of teratogenic fears should the woman become pregnant during the following menstrual cycle.

• *Prostaglandin Synthetase Inhibitors.* Mefanamic acid is the preferred choice of prostaglandin synthetase inhibitor. It not only reduces prostaglandin synthesis in the endometrium, but also binds to the prostaglandin receptors. Almost 75% of women treated with mefanamic acid experience 25% to 40% reduction in menstrual blood loss. Women with moderately severe HMB are, therefore, among the most satisfied with this treatment. Mefanamic acid also carries an additional benefit of reduction of dysmenorrhea, menstrual migraine, nausea and vomiting.

• *Oral Tranexamic Acid.* This anti-fibrinolytic agent is the first-line medical therapy for women with more severe HMB. It reduces menstrual blood loss by as much as 50% when used at 3 g/day for the first three days of menstruation. No increased risk of thromboembolic events has been associated with the use of tranexamic acid in this manner among young women.

• *Progestogen.* High dose progesterone (norethisterone 30 mg/day) during the acute phase of HMB is effective in arresting bleeding through multiple mechanisms of action. Progesterone stabilizes endometrium, reduces endometrial fibrinolysis by inhibiting release of tPA, and enhances vasoconstriction by increasing endometrial secretion of PG F2α, which, in turn promotes release of endothelin.

(ii) **Long-term Therapy for Chronic HMB.** The choice of either medical or surgical methods for long-term management of idiopathic HMB depends on the age and desire for fertility of the woman. There are non-hormonal and hormonal medical therapies.

• *Cyclic Progestogen.* Norethisterone, medroxyprogesterone and dydrogesterone are available oral progestogen. They suppress the endometrium and give rise to depleted glands lined by thin endometrium and decidualized stroma. When given at 5 mg/day from day-5 to day-25 of the menstrual cycle, norethistorone reduces menstrual blood loss by 30%. Given in this cyclic manner, norethisterone also regulates the onset of the next menstruation. In addition, there is a contraceptive effect on the treatment cycle. The main side effects of oral progesterone therapy are breast tenderness and swelling, acne, weight gain and bloating.

• *Continuous Progesterone Therapy.* This can be given in the form of oral tablets, long-term repeated intramuscular injections, or intrauterine progestogen releasing system. The resultant endometrial atrophy reduces the menstrual blood loss. Many women thus treated develop either irregular oligomenorrhea or amenorrhea. The other side effects are progesterone-related as seen with cyclic hormonal therapy. The endometrial changes are rapidly reversible upon withdrawal of treatment.

• *Combined Estrogen-Progestogen Therapy* in the form of oral contractive pills has been shown to reduce HMB by up to 50%

and is particularly useful in younger women who also desire contraception or regulation of irregular menstrual cycle. Its use in women above 40-years old is not contraindicated if she has no other risk factors for thromboembolism such as obesity, hypertension or cigarette smoking.

• *Danazol* used in low dose (200 mg/day) is well tolerated and has been reported to reduce HMB by up to 50% in short-term and oligomenorrhea or amenorrhea in continual usage.

• *GnRH Agonists*. Synthetic GnRH agonists induce a state of pituitary hypogonadism and amenorrhea. Its use in idiopathic HMB is limited by its hypo-estrogenic side effects.

• *Hysteroscopic Endometrial Surgery*. Surgical treatment for idiopathic HMB is appropriate for women who are no longer desired fertility, particularly if medical treatment is unsuccessful or intolerable.

Hysteroscopic endometrial surgery aims to reduce the thickness of the endometrium, the source of menstruation. In the endometrial resection technique, the endometrium is scraped out with a loop diathermy through a hysteroscopic resectoscope. The resected endometrium is removed through the cervix. Alternatively, endometrium ablation employs a number of possible physical modalities to destroy the endometrium. The first generation technique of roller ball diathermy has been replaced with the second generation impedance-controlled radiofrequency, microwave, thermal balloon, or free fluid hydrothermal techniques. Depending on the extent of endometrial resection or ablation, the patient may experience amenorrhea or oligomenorrhea. Regeneration of endometrium with recurrence of HMB may occur and repeated surgeries may be necessary. Approximately 20% of women treated with hysteroscopic resection or ablation eventually undergo hysterectomy.

Hysteroscopic endometrial surgery is a simple technique which can be performed as a day-case surgery with a short recovery time and low complication rate. The most common complication is uterine perforation which occurs in 1% of patient. Overall, 75% of women are satisfied with conservative hysteroscopic endometrial surgery.

• *Hysterectomy*. This is the permanent cure for HMB and has been shown to carry a patient satisfaction rate of more than 90%. It is a suitable treatment only if the patient has no desire for fertility. Also, hysterectomy is a major surgery associated with a small but definite risk of serious morbidity and mortality. Compared to abdominal hysterectomy, vaginal or laparoscopic hysterectomy has a shorter postoperative recovery time and is the preferred mode of surgery.

Illustration of Some Conditions that Cause HMB

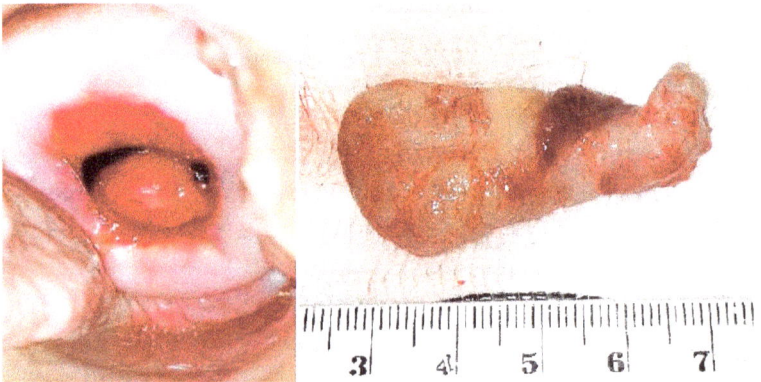

This woman complained of heavy menstrual bleeding for several months. In the most recent menstruation, the flow was extremely heavy and did not show any signs of abating after 10 days. On examination, her uterus was normal in size and a speculum examination demonstrated a cervical polyp seen the cervical os (panel on the left hand side). The entire polyp is shown in the panel on the right, after a polypectomy procedure was performed. The bleeding problem resolved.

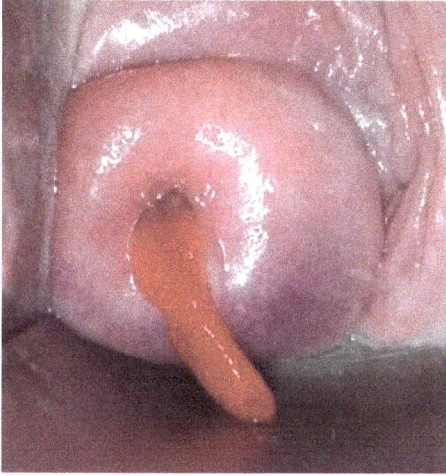

This 45-year-old woman complained of heavy menstrual bleeding for several months. The uterus was normal in size and a speculum examination demonstrated a tongue-like polyp protruding through the cervical os. Ultrasound scan confirmed that she had a large endometrial polyp, part of which presented as this "cervical polyp."

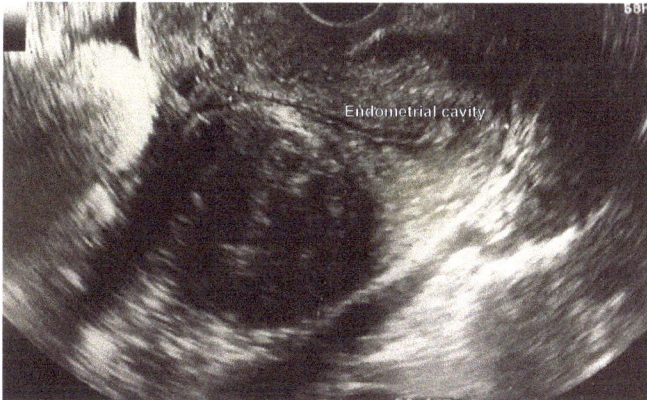

This 38-year-old woman complained of increasingly heavy menstrual bleeding in the past one year. The uterus was enlarged to 8-week gestation size. A pelvic ultrasound scan demonstrated a 6-cm fibroid extending into the endometrium — submucous fibroid. This is the commonest type of fibroid causing HMB.

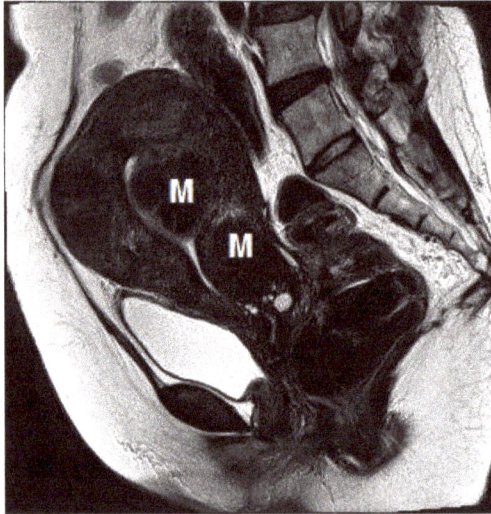

This 48-year-old woman complained of a 12-month history of heavy menstrual bleeding and was found to have a 14-week gestation size uterus. A pelvic MRI scan demonstrated two large submucous uterine fibroids (marked "M" in the photograph) distorting the endometrial cavity.

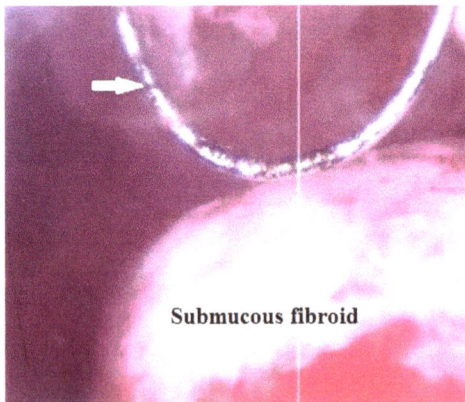

Submucous fibroid

This photograph shows the submucous fibroid treated with transcervical hysteroscopic resection. The white arrow identifies the cutting electric wire loop for fibroid resection. The same device is used for resecting endometrium for treatment of HMB without fibroids.

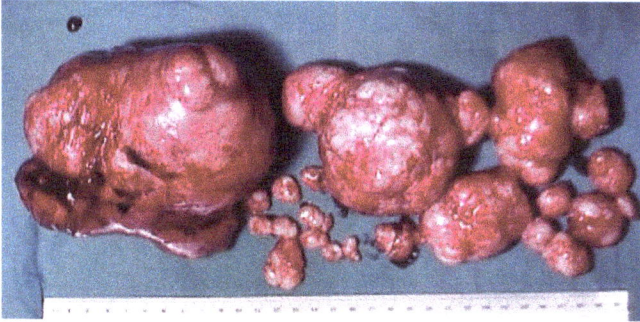

This 35-year-old woman experienced HMB that had become progressively unbearable. She was found to have an enlarged uterus from multiple fibroids. In view of her young age, she opted to undertake myomectomy surgery. This photograph shows multiple fibroids removed during the surgery.

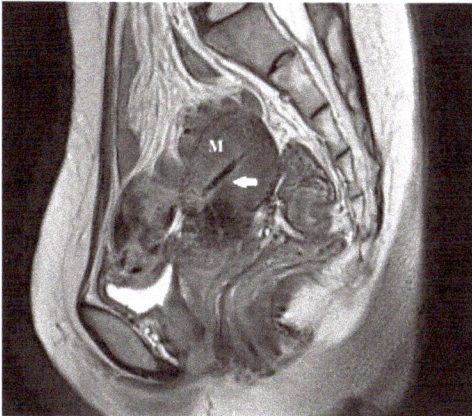

This 32-year-old woman experienced progressively worsening HMB with associated dysmenorrhea. This photograph of a section of T2 signal MR imaging study shows the loss of junctional zone between the endometrium (identified by the white arrow) and the myometrium (marked "M"), consistent with diagnosis of uterine adenomyosis.

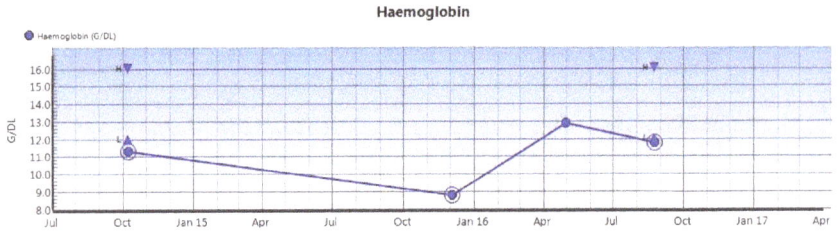

Haemoglobin

This chart shows the trend in serum hemoglobin level in a woman who complained of HMB. Medical therapy with oral tranexamic acid tablets during menstrual phase resulted in prompt return of hemoglobin level of 8.9 g/L in January 2016 to 13.0 g/L in May 2016. The slight decline in hemoglobin level in September 2016 highlights a problem of treatment compliance of long-term oral medication.

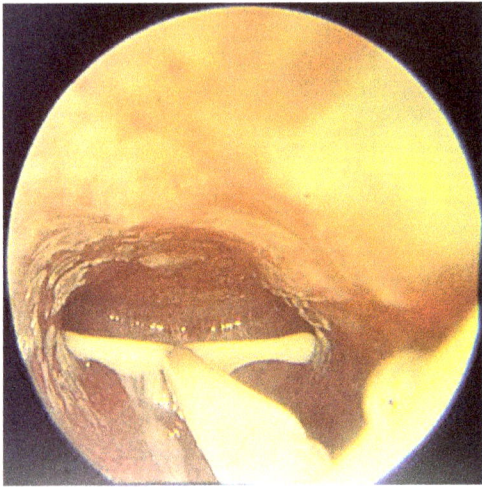

This photograph of hysteroscopy shows the atrophic endometrium following the use of levonorgestrel intrauterine delivery system (Mirena®). The woman was amenorrheic for 2 years.

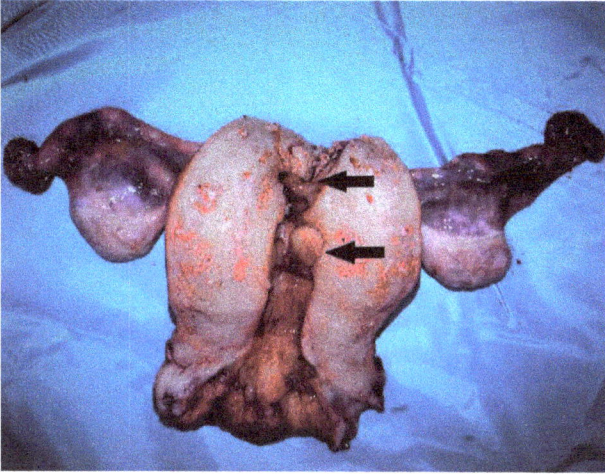

This photograph of a total hysterectomy and bilateral salpingo-oophorectomy shows an endometrial cancer (arrows). The 48-year-old patient presented with a 2-month history of prolonged and heavy menstrual bleeding.

CASE 7 — POST-COITAL BLEEDING

A 35-year-old para-2 woman complains of fresh vaginal bleeding after sexual intercourse.

- What is the common medical term for this complaint?
- What are the possible sources of this bleeding?
- What conditions may explain her symptoms?

What is the Common Medical Term for this Complaint?

In the absence of menstruation, any vaginal bleeding, either during or after sexual intercourse, is known as post-coital bleeding (PCB). Its prevalence among women in the reproductive life ranges from 0.7% to 9%. The reported prevalence is influenced by criteria used to define the condition, such as frequency and temporal relationship between the symptom and sexual intercourse. PCB is present with concomitant abnormal menstrual bleeding in 30% and dyspareunia in 15% of cases.

What are the Possible Sources of this Bleeding?

PCB may be uterine in origin, but most commonly, bleeding occurs from the cervix or vagina.

What Conditions may Explain her Symptoms?

Cancer, particularly cervical cancer, is the most feared condition that causes PCB. Cervical cancer is a rarity in women below 25-years old and these young patients should not be alarmed. Among older women investigated for PCB in British hospitals, cancer was found in 2.7% of the cases. However, as 10% to 30% of cervical carcinoma present with PCB, a much higher incidence of cervical cancer is found in women complaining of PCB in countries where cervical cancer screening is not available and where the prevalence of the cancer is high.

Other commonly encountered conditions among women complaining of PCB are genital tract infection (20%), cervical ectropion (15%) and cervical polyps (5%). No pathology was found in almost 45% of cases.

Based on the source of bleeding, conditions that may cause post-coital bleeding include:

(i) **Uterine Causes**
   - Endometrial polyps
   - Endometritis
   - Intrauterine contraceptive device (IUD)
   - Endometrial cancer

(ii) **Cervical Lesions**
   - Cervical ectropion
   - Cervicitis
   - Cervical polyp
   - Cervical carcinoma
   - Cervical warts

(iii) **Vaginal Lesions**
   - Vaginitis
   - Vaginal warts
   - Vaginal trauma
   - Vaginal carcinoma

Selected Condition

Cervical Ectropion (Cervical Eversion)

This physiological state of the cervix was previously known as cervical erosion. The misnomer carries a pathological connotation which prompted unwary physicians to initiate treatments unnecessarily.

The vaginal portion of the cervix is covered by columnar epithelium in the endocervical canal and squamous epithelium in the ectocervix. The two epithelia meet at the squamo-columnar junction (SCJ). In pre-pubertal adolescents, SCJ is located within the endocervix and is not visible on inspection during speculum examination of the cervix. The cervix is entirely covered by multi-layered squamous epithelium and it assumes a smooth and pale pink appearance.

With the surge of circulating estrogen during puberty and during pregnancy, the cervix grows in size. The external os becomes everted, and the relative change in location of SCJ to the exposed ectocervix gives rise to an apparent appearance of a red and soft tissue around the external os or a visual appearance of erosion. In effect, the red "erosion" is the appearance of normal single layer columnar epithelium of the lower portion of the endocervix.

Cervical ectropion evolves under the influence of an acidic environment of the vagina. The columnar epithelium undergoes squamous metaplasia. Mature metaplastic squamous epithelium is indistinguishable from original squamous epithelium and substantiated the old concept that the "erosion" has healed.

Matured squamous epithelium and columnar epithelium forms a new SCJ and the area of metaplastic squamous epithelium between the old and new SCJs is known to colposcopist as the transformation zone. This is the site where cervical pre-malignancy and invasive cancer develop.

Illustration of Some Conditions Encountered in Women Complaining of PCB

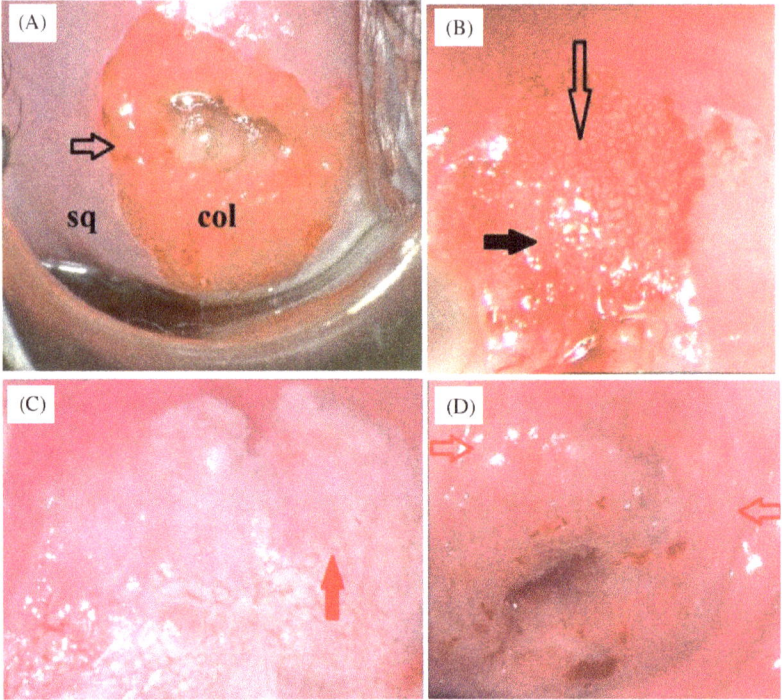

This panel of photographs shows the evolution of ectropion of the cervix in a 25-year-old woman. In panel (A), the ectropion shows a sharp demarcation between squamous epithelium (marked "sq") and columnar epithelium (marked "col"). The junction between them is known as squamo-columnar junction (SCJ, marked by the open arrow). In panel (B), the villous-like columnar structures get closer at the surface (marked by open arrow) and then become coalesced (marked by solid arrow). In panel (C), the squamous metaplasia forms a smooth and pearly white epithelium which is to be distinguished from aceto-white of pre-malignancy, and forms a new squamo-columar junction (marked by solid red arrow). Finally, squamous metaplasia completes the process of maturation as shown in panel (D). The original squamo-columnar junction is marked by open red arrows.

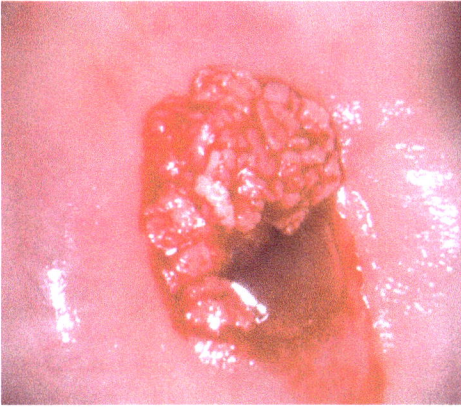

This photograph shows a tumor at the central portion of the cervix in a 30-year-old woman complaining of PCB for 2 weeks.

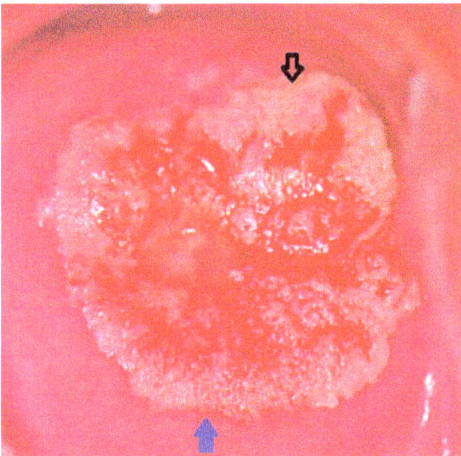

This 29-year-old woman complained of post-coital bleeding. The photograph shows a florid ectropion-like lesion. A cervical cytology was performed and it showed a high-grade squamous intraepithelial lesion. A colposcopy was performed. The blue arrow showed that the lesion had a slightly raised edge and an appearance of genital warts. The central portion of the lesion was hemorrhagic which was responsible for her symptom. The open black arrow identified an area of abnormal epithelium which was proven to be cervical intraepithelial neoplasia grade-3 on biopsy.

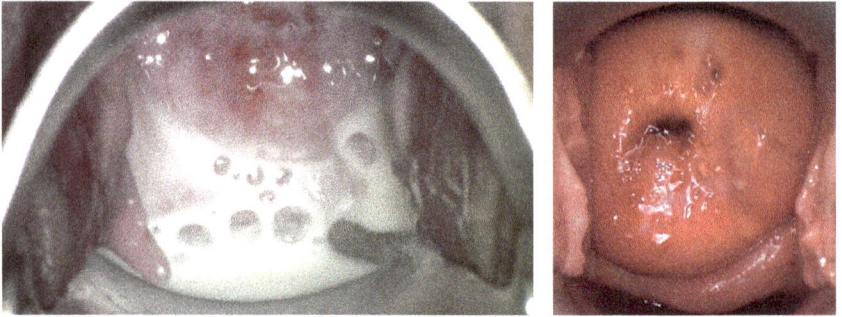

These photographs shows a case of chronic cervicitis in a 33-year-old woman who complained of bleeding of fresh blood during and after sexual intercourse. The panel on the left hand side shows a profuse vaginal discharge. After removing the discharge, it was evident that there was an inflammation involving the entire cervix as shown in the panel of the photographs on the right hand side.

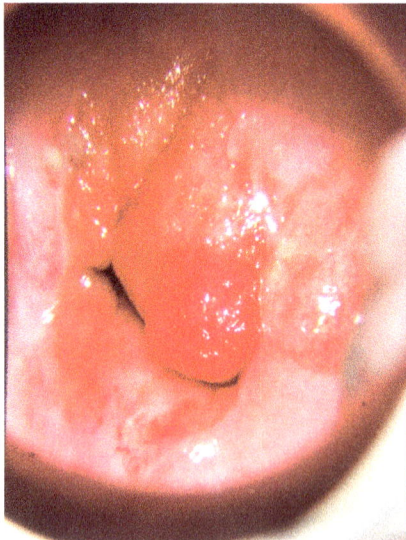

This photograph shows a sessile polyp at the periphery of an ectropion of the cervix in a 48-year-old woman who complained of light bleeding after sexual intercourse.

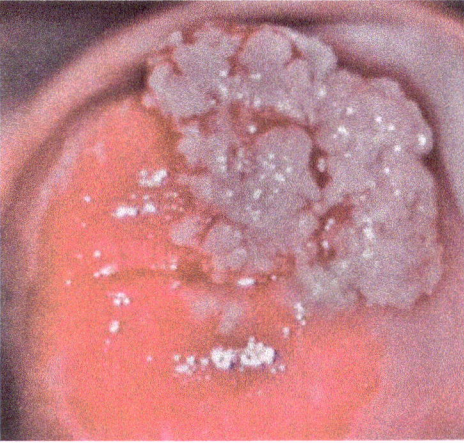

This 23-year-old woman complained of a short history of post-coital bleeding. This photograph shows that she had a large cervical condyloma. Isolated genital warts on the cervix are uncommon. Condyloma is more commonly encountered on the external genitalia.

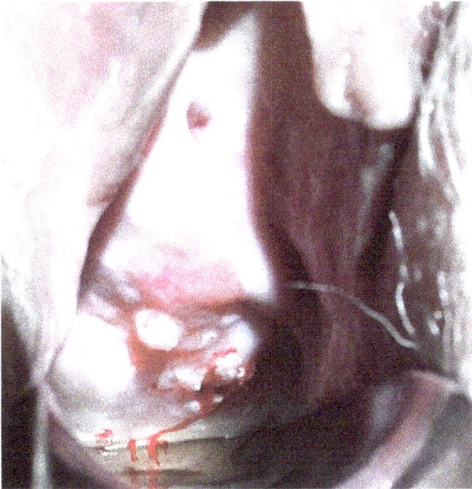

This 65-year-old woman complained of bleeding after sexual intercourse. The photograph shows a tumor on the anterior wall of the lower one third of the vagina.

CASE 8 — POSTMENOPAUSAL BLEEDING

A 60-year-old para-0 woman complains of vaginal bleeding for one week.

- How often does postmenopausal bleeding occur?
- What conditions may cause postmenopausal bleeding?
- How should postmenopausal bleeding be evaluated?

How Often does Postmenopausal Bleeding Occur?

Postmenopausal bleeding (PMB) is defined as spontaneous vaginal bleeding after established menopause. A life time risk of ever having an episode of PMB is approximately 10%, but the incidence of PMB decreases with increasing duration of menopause. A recent European study reported an incidence of 409/1000 women-year during the first 12 months of menopause and 42/1000 women-year among women who had menopause for more than 3 years.

What Condition may Cause Postmenopausal Bleeding?

The source of vaginal bleeding can be the genital tract or adjacent organs.

Genital Tract Bleeding

- Uterine corpus — Polyps; Endometritis; Endometrial hyperplasia; Endometrial carcinoma; Exogenous estrogen therapy; Tamoxifen therapy.

- Cervix — Polyps; Cervicitis; Carcinoma
- Vagina — Vaginitis; carcinoma
- Vulva — vulvitis; carcinoma
- Fallopian tube — Carcinoma
- Ovarian lesions — Carcinoma; Granulosa cell tumor

Non-genital Tract Bleeding

- Urinary bladder — Cystitis; Carcinoma
- Urethra — Caruncle
- Anus — Hemorrhoids; Carcinoma
- Colo-rectum — Hemorrhoids; Carcinoma

How should Postmenopausal Bleeding be Evaluated?

As endometrial cancer is predominantly a postmenopausal disease and 90% of endometrial cancer presents with uterine bleeding, all postmenopausal bleeding, however small quantity the bleeding may be, should be evaluated. Endometrial cancer is found in 5% (range 1% to 10%) and endometrial polyps in 10% of women investigated for PMB. Clinical examination will reveal lesions in the lower genital tract but further investigations with cervical cancer screening, pelvic ultrasound scan and endometrial biopsy are indicated.

The most informative investigation in evaluating uterine pathology in PMB is a pelvic ultrasound scan. Transvaginal ultrasound scan of the pelvis has a very high sensitivity in detecting ovarian and endometrial pathology. In postmenopausal women, the mean endometrial thickness measures 2.3 mm among women with no bleeding, 3.9 mm among women with PMB and 21 mm among women with endometrial carcinoma. Using an endometrial thickness of 5 mm as a cut-off value, the sensitivity and specificity of detecting endometrial carcinoma is 85% and 75%, respectively. The risk of endometrial carcinoma increases with increasing endometrial thickness: 4.6% for thickness less than 4 mm, 16% for thickness between 4–10 mm, and 55% for thickness between 10–15 mm. The negative predictive value is 99%.

Endometrial biopsy with an office procedure carries the same sensitivity as formal dilatation and curettage in detecting endometrial cancer and has been established to be the procedure of choice in pathological assessment of the endometrium in PMB. Women with ultrasound measurement of endometrial thickness less than 4 mm and have normal cervical cytology can be spared from an endometrial biopsy, unless PMB recurs. The absolute risk of endometrial cancer is 8% among women who have recurrent PMB within one year.

Hysteroscopy/Dilatation and Curettage. Women with PMB showing a thickened endometrium but normal endometrial biopsy should be further evaluated with hysteroscopy. Hysteroscopy allows a panoramic survey of the uterine cavity and is highly sensitive for the diagnosis of uterine polyps and submucous fibroids. Among women with PMB and thickened endometrium, hysteroscopy revealed polyps in 36%, fibroids in 15%, endometrial hyperplasia in 25%, and endometrial cancer in 10%. In contrast, in the absence of PMB, postmenopausal women with a thickened endometrium were found to have polyps in 67%, hyperplasia in 3%, and none for endometrial cancer.

Hysteroscopy permits polyps to be removed on their detection and areas of abnormal appearing endometrium to be assessed by directed biopsy. In the absence of macroscopic endometrial abnormality on hysteroscopy, dilatation and curettage should be performed.

Selected Disease

Endometrial Carcinoma

This is the most common malignancy in pelvic reproductive organs in developed countries and, in Singapore, the incidence trend has been rising during the last four decades. It accounted for 6% of all cancers in Singaporean women between 2009 and 2013. The age distribution of the women diagnosed with endometrial cancer was 16% below 45 years old, 30% between 45 and 54 years old, and 54% after 55 years old.

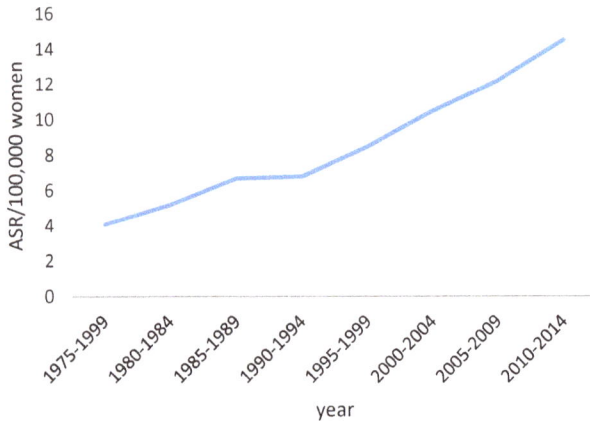

This chard shows the trend of age-standardized incidence rate (ASR) of endometrial carcinoma in Singapore from 1975 to 2014.

Approximately 90% of endometrial cancer manifest with abnormal uterine bleeding: menorrhagia, polymenorrhagia, and PMB. In cases of advanced endometrial cancer, especially patients with uterine papillary serous or clear cell histology type, there may be other symptoms such as abdominal pain and bloating, genital discharge, weight loss or change in bladder or bowel habits.

The risk of endometrial cancer increases by 2–3 folds in women with obesity, nulliparity, PCOS, hypertension, diabetes mellitus, and breast cancer. In postmenopausal women, history of early menarche or late menopause, and use of tamoxifen and unopposed estrogen replacement therapy are known risk factors for endometrial cancer. Among women with a family history of hereditary non-polyposis colonic cancer (HNPCC), where there is an autosomal dominant germline mutation in DNA mismatch repair (MMR) genes (*MSH1*, *MSH2*, *MSH6*), there is a 40–60% risk of endometrial cancer by the age of 70 years old. HNPCC accounts for 9% of patients who have a diagnosis of endometrial cancer below the age of 50 years, compared to a baseline population risk of 1.5% at the same age. It is noteworthy that 1% of HNPCC has endometrial or ovarian cancer diagnosed first as the sentinel cancer.

Conversely, women who have consumed combined estrogen-progestogen contraceptive pills for more than 12 months or who are on estrogen-progestogen replacement therapy after menopause experience a 50% reduction in the risk of endometrial cancer.

By histology classification, more than 80% of endometrial carcinomas are type I or endometrioid adenocarcinoma, often found in association with atypical endometrial hyperplasia. Its etiology is attributable to unopposed estrogen stimulation. Type II endometrial cancers are thought to be estrogen independent, occurring in older women, with high-grade histology types such as uterine papillary serous or clear cell adenocarcinoma. These cancers are driven by mutated P53 oncogene.

Diagnosis of endometrial cancer is based on office procedure of endometrial sampling or biopsy, or a formal hysteroscopy and dilation and curettage. Ultrasound scan of the pelvis may demonstrated a thickened endometrium and is particularly informative in postmenopausal women where normal endometrial thickness should be less than 3 mm. Pelvic magnetic resonance imaging (MRI) study may demonstrate the depth of myometrial invasion, cervical stromal invasion and extrauterine and peritoneal lymph node metastasis.

The stage of endometrial cancer is based on surgico-pathological assessment of tissues in total hysterectomy, bilateral salpingo-oophorectomy and pelvic and para-aortic lymphadenectomy. Because of the abnormal bleeding pattern, two thirds of endometrial cancer are diagnosed at FIGO stage-I.

Management of endometrial carcinoma is primarily by surgery which includes an abdominal exploration, obtaining

FIGO Staging Classification of Endometrial Carcinoma

Stage	Criteria
I	Tumor confined to uterine corpus
IA	Tumor confined to the uterus, no or < ½ myometrial invasion
IB	Tumor confined to the uterus, > ½ myometrial invasion
II	Cervical stromal invasion, but not beyond uterus
III	Tumor involving uterine adnexal tissue or vagina or retroperitoneal lymph nodes
IIIA	Tumor invades serosa or adnexa
IIIB	Vaginal and/or parametrial involvement
IIIC1	Pelvic node involvement
IIIC2	Para-aortic involvement
IV	Tumor involving distant metastasis
IVA	Tumor invasion bladder and/or bowel mucosa
IVB	Distant metastases including abdominal metastases and/or inguinal lymph nodes

abdominal washings for cytology, total hysterectomy, bilateral salpingo-oophorectomy, biopsy of any suspicious lesions, and pelvic and para-aortic lymphadenectomy. Omentectomy is also indicated for papillary serous or clear cell carcinoma. The surgery can be performed via laparotomy, laparoscopic or robot-assisted surgery.

Post-surgery adjuvant therapy is recommended according to risk stratification for relapse cancer.

1. **Low Risk**: no adjuvant therapy
   - Stage IA cancer
2. **Moderate Risk**: external and/or vaginal brachytherapy
   - IBG1, G2 or
   - Presence of any two of the following three risk factors: grade 3 histology, age over 60 years, or >1/2 thickness of myometrium invasion

3. **High Risk**: radiation and/or chemotherapy and pelvic radiotherapy
    - All G3 or Stage II and above
    - Serous, Clear cell carcinoma

In exceptional situation, young women who want to preserve fertility, hormonal therapy with either high dose medroxyprogesterone or GnRH analogue may be attempted. The tumor characteristic must fulfill the following criteria:

- Stage I type-I cancer with no myometrial invasion,
- No lymphovascular space involvement
- Tumor histology belongs to FIGO grade-1
- Negative peritoneal cytology
- Complete informed consent, including commitment for close follow up.

Illustration of Some Conditions that can Cause PMB

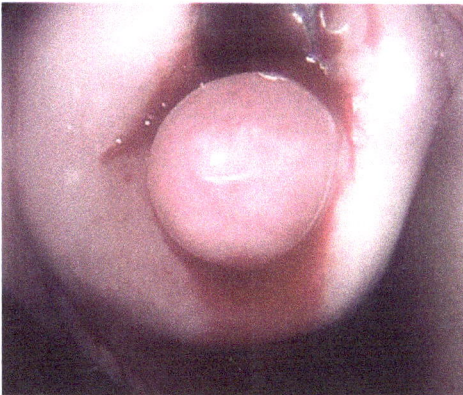

This elderly woman complained of intermittent scanty blood staining on the undergarment. Symptomatic review was otherwise negative. Examination showed a polyp on the cervix.

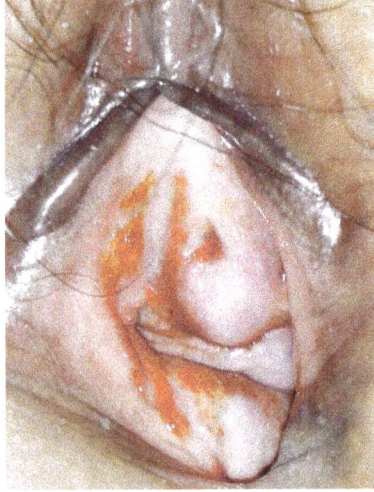

This elderly woman complained of scanty bleeding on attending to toilet. She was found to have severe atrophic vaginitis which bled on wiping with tissue paper.

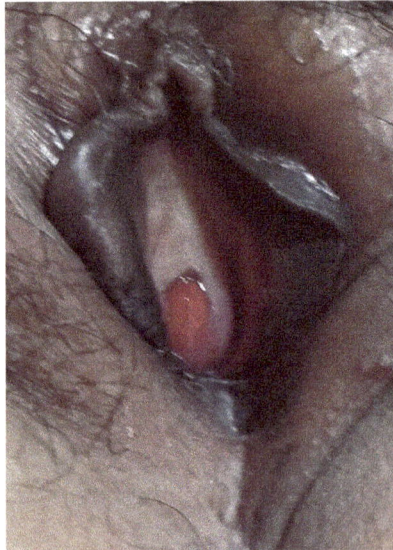

This elderly woman complained of small quantity of fresh looking blood on the underwear. She was found to have a prolapsed urethral meatus mucosa (caruncle). The lesion resolved on topical estrogen application.

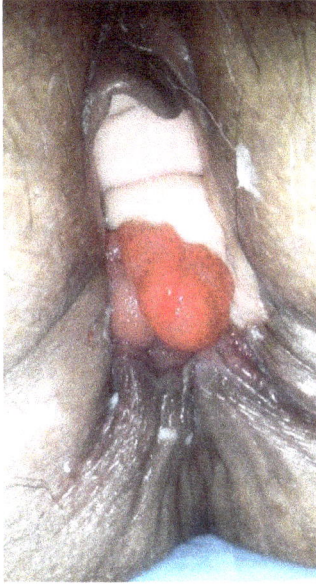

This 85-year-old woman complained of increasing vagina discharge for two years. The discharge became blood stained for the recent three months. This photograph shows that she had a vulvar carcinoma involving the perineum and the introitus of the vagina.

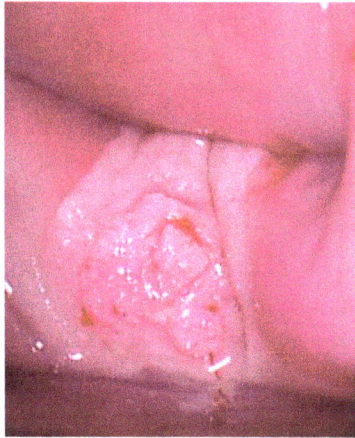

This 55-year-old woman complained of a 3-month history of PMB was found to have an area of contact bleeding. This photograph of a colposcopy examination shows a vagina cancer with contact bleeding.

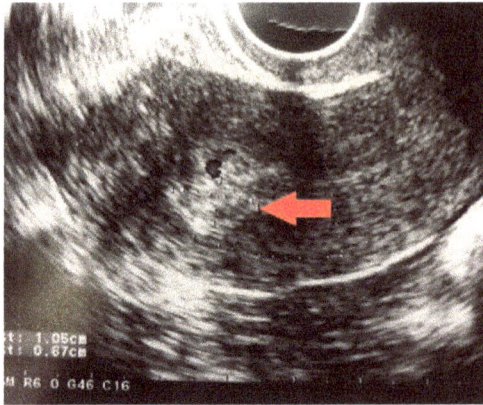

Transvaginal ultrasound scan has a very high sensitivity for detection of endometrial cancer. This photograph of ultrasound scan of the uterus shows a focus endometrial thickening (marked by the red arrow) in a woman complaining of PMB. Histopathology of an endometrial biopsy confirm a carcinoma of the endometrium.

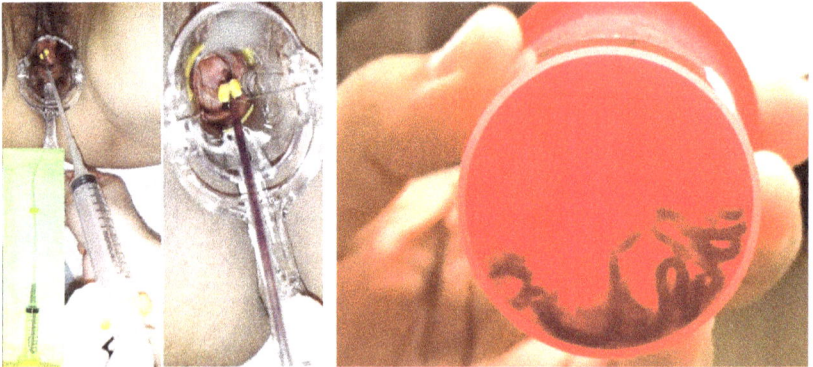

This panel of photographs shows an endometrial sampling device (left bottom insert). The device was introduced into the uterine cavity (left panel) and suction from the syringe aspirated a sample of endometrium (right panel). This office procedure has largely replaced formal dilatation curettage under general anesthesia for evaluation of endometrial pathology.

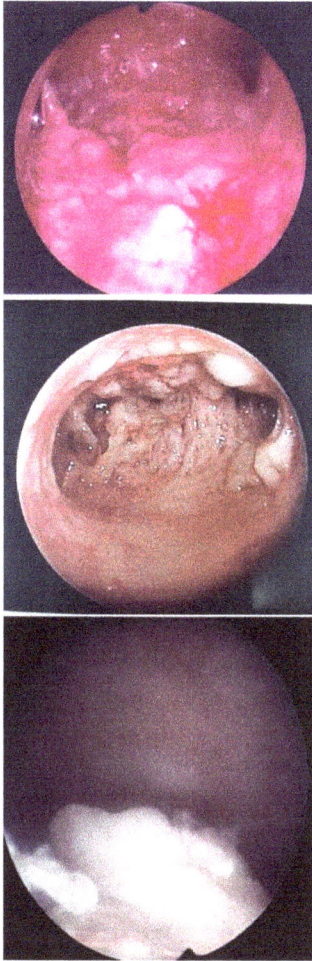

This panel of photographs shows the pathologic appearance of endometrium on hysteroscopy. Hysteroscopy has a high sensitivity in detection of uterine polyp and fibroids but a low sensitivity in distinguishing endometrial hyperplasia from invasive endometrial cancer.

The photograph at the top of the panel shows endometrial hyperplasia with cobblestone appearance on hysteroscopy.

The photograph at middle shows irregular and nodular endometrial appearance of an early endometrial carcinoma.

The photograph at the bottom shows a polypoidal tumor of endometrial carcinoma.

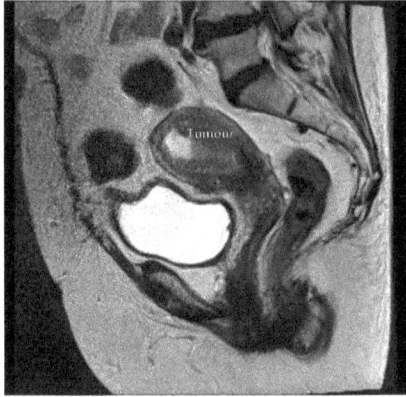

This photograph of a magnetic resonance (MR) image (T-2 signal) of sagittal plane of the pelvis shows an endometrial cancer in the fundal portion of the uterine cavity.

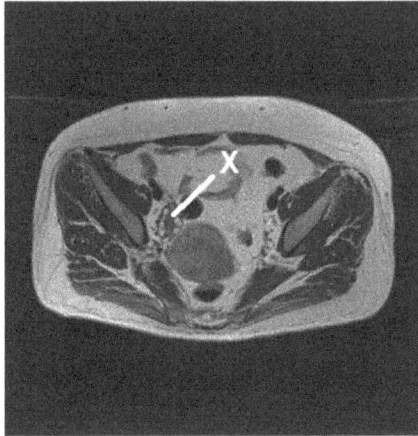

This MRI image (T-2 signal) shows a polycystic ovary (marked "X") in a 30-year-old woman with endometrial carcinoma. Chronic anovulation from polycystic ovarian syndrome is the commonest cause of endometrioid adenocarcinoma in women below the age of 40 years.

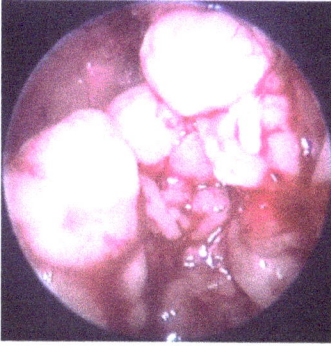

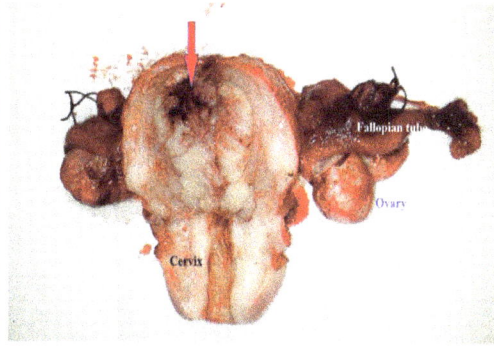

The photograph on the left shows a tumor revealed on hysteroscopy in a woman complaining of PMB. This cancerous lesion was treated with a total hysterectomy, bilateral salpingo-oophorectomy, the mainstay treatment of endometrial carcinoma. In this photograph of surgical specimen, which was cut opened to show the tumor (marked by the red arrow) which occupied the entire uterine cavity, and the tumor has reached the level of the internal os of the cervix.

CASE 9 — DYSMENORRHEA

A 25-year-old woman seeks treatment for a severe lower abdominal pain during her menstruation.

- What is known as primary and secondary dysmenorrhea?
- What is the etiology and treatment of primary dysmenorrhea?
- What conditions may cause secondary dysmenorrhea?

What is Known as Primary and Secondary Dysmenorrhea?

Dysmenorrhea refers to lower abdominal pain associated with menstruation. It may radiate to the back or down into the legs and is commonly described as cramping or "labor-like." There may be associated symptoms, including headache, nausea and vomiting, diarrhea, bloating, mood change, and fatigue. Almost 90% of adolescents and 25% of adult women experience dysmenorrhea. In these cases, 50% has debilitating pain, 50% reports absenteeism from school or work, and 20% requires regular medical consultation and treatment.

Clinically, dysmenorrhea is classified into Primary and Secondary Dysmenorrhea. Primary dysmenorrhea is idiopathic, in contrast to secondary dysmenorrhea which is dysmenorrhea associated with organic disorders of the uterus or medical conditions.

The diagnosis of dysmenorrhea relies on the history of pelvic pain specifically related to menstruation. Distinct clinical features of primary and secondary dysmenorrhea are summarized below:

Clinical Features	Types of Dysmenorrhea	
	Primary	Secondary
Onset from menarche	Within 6 months	Anytime
Onset from menstruation	At starting	Before or at starting
Age at onset	Adolescence	Anytime, most commonly 30–45 years old
Duration of pain	24–48 hours	Up to entire menstruation
Presence of other gynecological symptoms	None	Common, e.g. dyspareunia, vaginal discharge, heavy menstrual bleeding, intermenstrual bleeding, post-coital bleeding
Pelvic examination	Normal	Often abnormal (normal pelvic examination does not exclude secondary dysmenorrhea)
Ovulatory cycle	Always	Not necessary
Resolve after pregnancy	Often	No
Response to NSAIDS or OCP	Good	Unreliable

The definitive diagnosis of primary or secondary dysmenorrhea is determined by whether a pelvic disease is detected on thorough clinical examinations and on investigations. Pelvic ultrasound scan is the most useful investigational tool for detecting conditions causing secondary dysmenorrhea. Other investigations may include MR imaging, hysteroscopy and laparoscopy, and appropriate histological and bacteriological examination of the endometrium or pelvic organs.

What is the Etiology and Treatment of Primary Dysmenorrhea?

Etiology

Uterus is a contractile organ with myometrial fibers arranged in layers separated by junctional zone which is best delineated on MR imaging. During the necrosis and sloughing phase of menstruation, elevation of both prostaglandins F2α and E_2, and endothelin induces increased uterine contractility. Vasopressin also presents as a potent uterine constrictor.

Two pathological changes in the uterus are evident in some women experiencing dysmenorrhea. Firstly, there are structural changes in myometrial orientation and thickening of the junctional zones. Secondly, a higher level of PGF2α, PG E_2, endothelin and vasopressin in menstrual blood is detected in women experiencing dysmenorrhea compared to women without dysmenorrhea. The resultant hypercontractility and increased muscular tone of the uterus, and vasoconstriction give rise to uterine ischemic pain, or "uterine angina" of dysmenorrhea.

Primary dysmenorrhea is more commonly encountered in girls or women with an early menarche before the age of 12 years. Other factors associated with increased risk of primary dysmenorrhea include increased body weight or obesity or attempts to lose weight (regardless of body weight), cigarette smoking, and mental state of stress, anxiety and depression.

Treatment of Primary Dysmenorrhea

There is no effective permanent cure of primary dysmenorrhea. The primary objective of treatment is to reduce the pain and to improve the quality of life of the women. Assuring the girls that primary dysmenorrhea does not carry serious pelvic pathology and that it has a good prognosis with spontaneous resolution, in particular after a pregnancy, may be sufficient to allay the anxiety and thus improve their ability to cope with mild primary dysmenorrhea.

In more severe cases, non-steroidal anti-inflammatory drugs (NSAIDS) are efficacious in more than 80% of cases and are the treatment of first choice. The effectiveness appears to be equal for all the available prostaglandin synthetase inhibitors such as mefenamic acid, diclofenac acid, and naproxen sodium, and COX-2 inhibitors such as etoricoxib and celecoxib. Paracetamol is as effective as NSAIDS and the efficacy seems to be further enhanced by combining with caffeine. Aspirin is not as effective as NSAIDS.

Combined oral estrogen-progestogen contraceptive pills are widely used for treatment of both primary and secondary dysmenorrhea. This is particularly indicated if the woman also requires contraception. Significant pain relief can be achieved in almost 50% of women with either second or third generation combined oral contraceptive pills. Adverse side effects such as nausea and vomiting, headache, and weight gain are the main barriers to the use of this line of therapy.

Non-pharmacological approach with high frequency transcutaneous electric nerve stimulation, but not acupuncture, is more effective than placebo in lessening primary dysmenorrhea.

What Conditions may Cause Secondary Dysmenorrhea?

The common causes of secondary dysmenorrhea are uterine adenomyosis, endometriosis, fibroids, pelvic inflammatory disease (PID), endometrial polyps, intrauterine contraceptive device (IUCD), cervical stenosis (e.g. after uterine or cervical surgery), congenital malformations (e.g. imperforated hymen), and ovarian cysts or tumors.

Selected Diseases

1. Uterine Adenomyosis

The exact incidence of uterine adenomyosis is unknown. Among women who experience difficulty of conceiving, dysmenorrhea or heavy menstrual bleeding, the prevalence of adenomyosis has been reported to be approximately 50%.

The pathology of uterine adenomyosis is characterized by extension of endometrial glandular and stromal tissues for more than 2.5 mm below the endomyometrial junction in low-power field on light microscopy. It may occur diffusely across the entire body of the uterus, the entire thickness of uterine wall, or limited to focal areas to form nodules known as adenomyomas. There is hyperplasia of junctional zone of exceeding 12 mm in thickness on MR imaging. Uterine adenomyosis may co-exist with pelvic endometriosis in more than 50% of cases.

Clinical manifestation of uterine adenomyosis varies from no symptom to severe dysmenorrhea and heavy menstrual bleeding. The symptomatology is modified by any co-existing endometriosis. Uterine adenomyosis may present with infertility or early pregnancy loss from anatomy abnormalities and associated angiogenesis aberration in junctional zone. During clinical examination, the uterus with diffuse adenomyosis exhibits a firm or hard consistency and the volume of the uterus assumes a globular-shape enlargement. On the other hand, adenomyomas are found as an irregularly enlarged uterus. In the absence of acute inflammation during menstrual phase, adenomyosis is typically not tender on clinical palpation. Without pelvic endometriosis, or after adequate treatment of endometriosis, uterine adenomyosis is not associated with dyspareunia.

The most useful investigations for adenomyosis are transvaginal ultrasound scan (TVS) and MR imaging. The TVS features of adenomyosis include loss of distinction of the endometrial-myometrial junction, asymmetry in the myometrial thickness between anterior and posterior uterine walls, subendometrial myometrial striations, detection of myometrial cysts or fibrosis, and heterogeneous myometrial echotexture. The sensitivity of TVS for detection of adenomyosis is 80%, but the specificity is about 50%. The performance of TVS is highly operator-dependent compared to MR imaging. Thickening of junctional zone beyond 12 mm on T2-weighted MR imaging is the most suggestive sign of adenomyosis. However, the diagnostic MR features of adenomyosis are detection of submucosal microcysts of islets of the ectopic endometrium with cystic glandular dilatation, and adenomyoma of focal consolidation of adenomyotic glands within myometrium. Microcysts are identifiable in 50% and adenomyoma in 30% of cases of adenomyosis. Combining the suggestive and definitive signs, MR imaging carries a sensitivity of 80% and specificity of 90% for uterine adenomyosis.

2. Endometriosis

This condition is characterized by development of endometrium-like tissue outside uterine cavity. It affects 10% of women in the general population and is diagnosed in more than 50% of women experiencing subfertility. It is second only to uterine fibroids as the commonest cause of major surgeries in women below the age of 45 years. Clinical manifestation of endometriosis typically presents as secondary dysmenorrhea initially and evolving progressively into chronic pelvic pain even in the absence of menstruation. There may be associated anal pain or tenesmus, bleeding per rectum, or hematuria. Dyspareunia is also present in 50% of women when endometriosis causes ovarian endometriomas or involves the Pouch of Douglas and uterosacral ligaments. Acute exacerbation of pelvic pain occurs if endometrioma leaks or ruptures. In general, pain of endometriosis occurs only in women of reproductive age when estrogenic effect is evident or in postmenopausal women who receives hormone replacement therapy.

The pathogenesis of endometriosis is complex and is not fully understood. It is believed to involve several mechanisms operating either singly or in combination.

(i) Transportation of shed endometrial tissues to the pelvic structures in retrograde flow of menstrual blood via the fallopian tubes. This hypothesis is supported by experiments in animals. Women with endometriosis, compared to those without endometriosis, are known to have higher intrauterine pressure and hypotonia of fallopian tubes. The resultant pressure gradient facilitates retrograde flow of the menstrual blood. It also explains the higher frequency of endometriosis involvement in gravity-dependent areas of the pelvis as compared with other anatomical sites.

(ii) Lymphatic dissemination of endometrial cells which explains the occurrence of endometriosis remote from the pelvis.

(iii) Coelomic metaplasia into endometrial-like tissue

(iv) Immunological changes in the peritoneal fluid which produces a peritoneal permissive environment for proliferation of ectopic endometrial tissues. Most notably, the macrophages are found to show an increase in immunosuppressive activities while the population of T-killer cells and natural killer cells is decreased.

(v) Biochemical changes which promotes proliferation of endometriotic tissues: there is a change in cytokine milieu rich in vascular endothelial growth factors which promote neo-angiogenesis, and, within the ectopic endometrial cells, there is an increase in aromatase activity which perpetuates the estrogen-dependent proliferation and progression of the disease.

(vi) Within the endometriotic cells, there are some somatic genetic aberrations which interfere with the normal regulation of cell proliferation.

Ectopic endometrium is responsive to endogenous and exogenous estrogen and progestogen. During the reproductive life, the ectopic endometrium exhibits cyclic cellular changes identical to the eutopic endometrium. During the menstrual phase, the increased secretion of prostaglandins and other cytokines in the ectopic endometrium results in the development of pelvic pain. More importantly, the cyclic deposition of hemorrhage at the site of the ectopic endometrium induces intense local inflammatory reactions, hemosiderin deposition, tissue fibrosis and scar formation and development of endometriomas. Endometriomas on the ovary are typically known as chocolate cysts to describe the chocolate appearance of altered blood within the cysts. These complications of endometriosis may implicate the adjacent organs causing bowel obstruction, ureteric obstruction, and bleeding from the bladder or bowels.

Diagnosis of endometriosis and adenomyosis is based on evaluation of clinical history and examination. Pelvic ultrasound scan may demonstrate endometriomas or adenomyomas. An elevation of serum CA125 level rules in the diagnosis of endometriosis. The diagnosis is confirmed on laparoscopy. If biopsy of endometriosis tissue is taken, histological examination reveals typical endometrial glands and stroma. For documentation and planning of treatment strategy, the extent of endometriosis is classified into minimal, mild, moderate and severe stages as originally devised by the American Society for Reproductive Medicine. Quantitative valuation of endometriosis is also performed with an Additive Diameter of Implants score which sums the diameters of all implants on laparoscopy. Neither of these classifications, however, correlates with the prognosis of subfertility treatment or the severity of pain a woman suffers.

The management of endometriosis is guided by the patient's goals of treatment: control of pelvic pain, treatment of subfertility, excision of large endometriomas, or correction of visceral or ureteric obstructions. The currently available medical and surgical options for pain management are summarized below:

Extent of Endometriosis	Treatment Option
Minimal	• Analgesic, e.g. NSAIDs • Hormonal, e.g. OCP, Progestin
Mild	• Analgesic, e.g. NSAIDs • Hormonal, e.g. OCP, Progestin • Laparoscopic ablation surgery
Moderate	• Laparoscopic excision with or without adjunctive hormonal therapy e.g. OCP, Progestin, GnRH analogs
Severe	• Surgical/Robotic excision with adjunctive hormonal therapy, e.g. OCP, Progestin, GnRH analogs • Hysterectomy and oophorectomies

Medical treatment is the first-line approach to pain control in endometriosis:

Types of Agent	Route of Administration	Mechanism of Action	Common Side Effects
NSAIDs	Oral	Prostaglandin synthetase inhibition	Gastric adverse effects
Combined estrogen-progestogen pills	Oral	Decidualization and endometrial atrophy	Nausea and vomiting, weight gain, headache
Progestogen	• Oral • Intramuscular • Intrauterine	Decidualization and endometrial atrophy	Nausea and vomiting, weight gain, menstrual changes
Anti-progestogen	Oral	Progestogen withdrawal effect; Inhibition of steroid-genesis	Androgenic side effects and hypoestrogenism
Danazol	Oral	Suppression of LH surge, raised free testosterone	Hirsutism, acne, deepening of voice
GnRH agonists	• Intranasal • Intramuscular • Subcutaneous	Down regulation of pituitary-ovarian axis	Hot flush, vaginal dryness, reduced libido, mood swings and depression, headache, bone loss
Aromatase inhibitors	Oral	Inhibit estrogen synthesis	Vaginal dryness, bone loss

Apart from NSAIDs which are prostaglandin synthetase inhibitors, all the other therapeutic agents manipulate the estrogen and progesterone effects in the endometrial cells. All these preparations are shown to be superior to placebo or no treatment in the efficacy of pain relief. The efficacy between the preparations seems to be similar, but the profile of adverse side effects is reflective of their mechanisms of action. As the disease runs a chronic course throughout the reproductive age of the woman, the prevalence and severity of adverse side effects become the fundamental guiding principle for selecting the therapeutic agent. Hormonal therapy has an advantage over analgesics as the period of pain control may extend for months beyond the treatment duration. The prolonged lifespan of the intrauterine levanorgetrel delivery system (Mirena) allows continual symptom control for five years.

Laparoscopy is the most common surgery performed for the diagnosis and treatment of endometriosis. Medical treatment of endometriomas is ineffective. They should be treated by definitive surgical excision which is proven superior to aspiration or drainage procedures. Laparoscopic ablation of mild to moderately severe endometriosis and excision of the more severe infiltrative endometriosis are effective treatment for pelvic pain in more than 60% of cases. Other surgical approaches include robotic surgery and laparotomy. The recurrence rates of endometriosis and pain after initial treatment are high, ranging from 20% at one year to more than 50% at five years of follow up. In term of pain control, the success rate of surgery is similar to medical treatment. For these reasons, surgery for pain control is indicated only if medical therapy has failed. Repeated surgery for recurring pelvic pain is undesirable and should be avoided as surgery carries a definite morbidity rate. Hysterectomy and bilateral salpingo-oophorectomy provides a permanent cure of endometriosis but is a surgery of the last resort for women who have intractable pain and who no longer desire to bear children.

Illustration of Some Conditions that Cause Dysmenorrhea

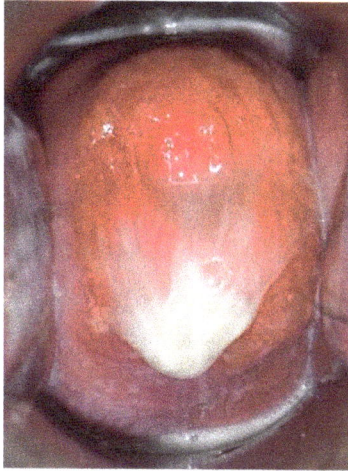

A 28-year-old woman with a recent onset of dysmenorrhea (secondary dysmenorrhea) was found to have an acute cervicitis with muco-purulent discharge. She has tender uterus on bimanual palpation and a clinical diagnosis of pelvic inflammatory disease.

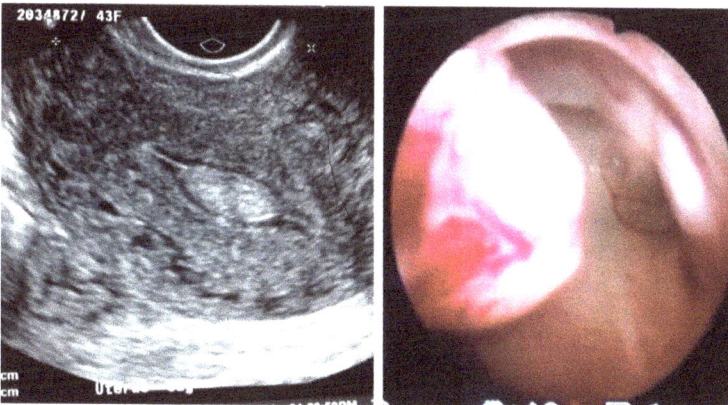

The panel of photographs on the left shows an ultrasound scan of a uterine polyp. The right panel shows a submucous fibroid on hysteroscopy. These two patients were investigated for secondary dysmenorrhea.

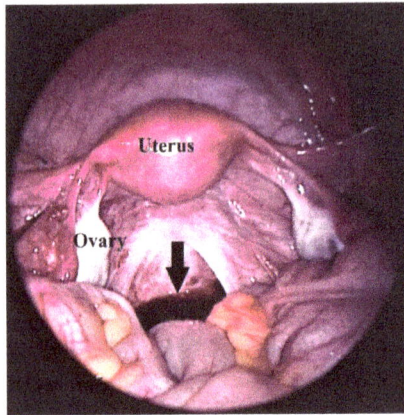

This photograph of a laparoscopy shows a normal pelvis with retrograde menstruation: the black arrow points to the menstrual blood in the Pouch of Douglas.

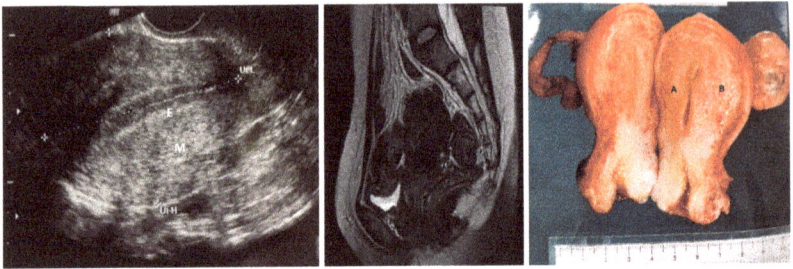

The panel of photographs above shows the pathology in a 48-year-old woman with increasing severity of secondary dysmenorrhea. She was found to have an enlarged uterus and a clinical diagnosis of uterine adenomyosis. An ultrasound scan of the uterus (left panel) shows an enlarged uterus with asymmetrical thickening of myometrium (marked "M") consistent with adenomyosis. MR imaging (central panel) shows a T-2 signal sagittal section of the uterus. The thickened junctional zone between endometrium and myometrium is an indication of adenomyosis. The woman had been treated with a variety of medications, including progestogen and intrauterine levonorgestrel delivery system. She opted for a total hysterectomy. The surgical specimen (right panel) shows normal myometrium (marked "A") in the anterior wall and adenomyosis (marked "B") in the posterior wall of the uterus. The uterine wall with adenomyosis was more than twice the thickness of the normal myometrium in this photograph.

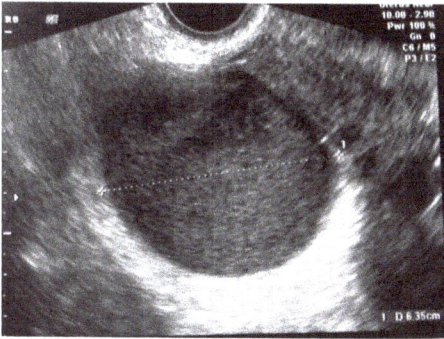

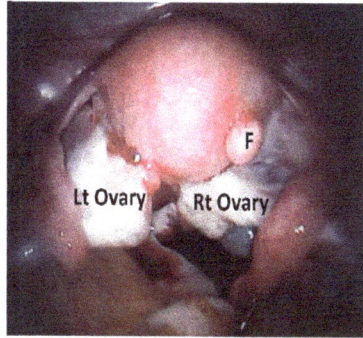

This 30-year-old nulliparous woman was investigated for secondary dysmenorrhea. The left panel shows a homogenous echogenic ovarian cyst of 6.3 cm in diameter on the left ovary. The feature was typical of an ovarian endometrioma. The diagnosis was confirmed on a laparoscopy as shown in the right panel of the photograph. The left ovary was densely adherent to the posterior surface of the uterus and was in a "kissing" relationship with the right ovary where a smaller endometrioma was also seen.

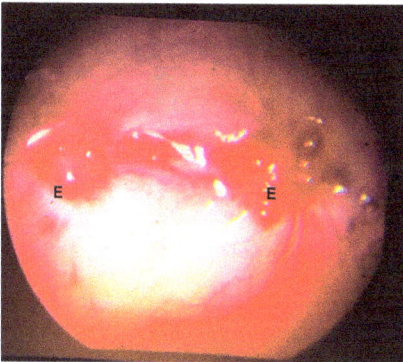

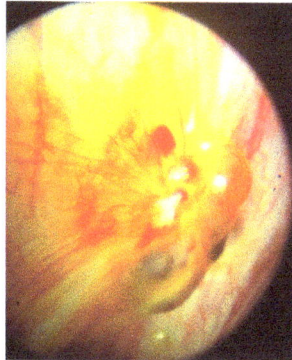

These photographs of laparoscopy show deposits of endometriosis on the peritoneum. The left panel shows fresh endometrium-like tissues with marked neovascular formation and inflammation (marked "E"). The right panel shows long-lasting peritoneal endometriosis with tissue hemosiderin deposits and marked fibrosis. Apart from dysmenorrhea, these patients experience dyspareunia.

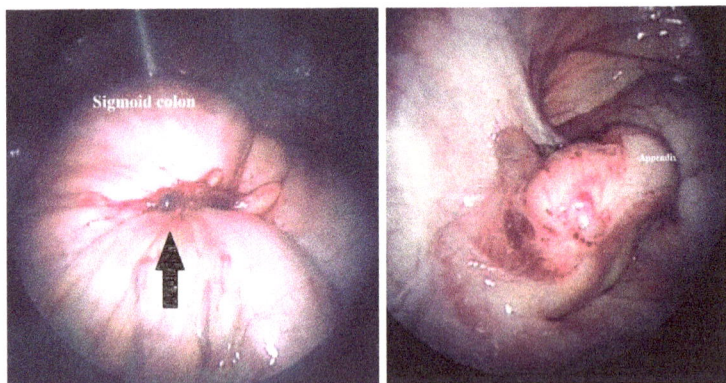

This 40-year-old woman complained of dysmenorrhea, dyspareunia, tenesmus and dychezia. The laparoscopic photograph on the left shows endometriosis on the sigmoid colon causing stenosis of the colon. The right panel of the photograph shows endometriosis deposits on the appendix.

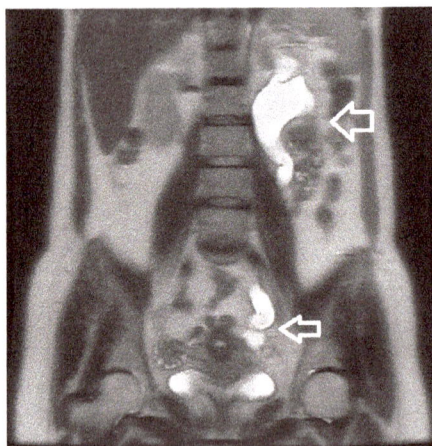

This 36-year-old woman had been treated for endometriosis for a number of years. In a new series of investigations for exacerbation of her symptoms, a MR imaging study revealed a gross hydroureter and hydronephrosis (marked arrows in the photograph). The ureter was implicated in deep infiltrative endometriosis in the parametrium. This patient underwent a total hysterectomy, resection of deep infiltrative endometriosis and re-implantation of the ureter.

CASE 10 — DYSPAREUNIA

A 28-year-old woman complains of painful sexual intercourse.

- What is the difference between dyspareunia and vaginismus?
- What conditions may cause dyspareunia?
- How is vaginismus treated?

What is the Difference between Dyspareunia and Vaginismus?

Dyspareunia refers to experience of pain in the vulva, vagina or pelvis during sexual intercourse. The pain may be experienced during vaginal penetration, during vaginal intercourse, or immediately after sexual intercourse. Clinically, dyspareunia is classified by the site of pain into superficial and deep dyspareunia. The prevalence of dyspareunia in the community is estimated at between 1% and 9%.

Vaginismus is a condition in which, despite the woman's expressed wish, vaginal penetration of penis, a finger and/or any object is unsuccessfully difficult over a persistent period of time. Although classified under dyspareunia, vaginismus may not be necessarily associated with pain. Vaginismus is a syndrome characterized by anxiety, fear, anticipation or actual experience of pain and involuntary pelvic muscle contraction. It leads to avoidance of sexual intercourse. Primary vaginismus refers to onset of the condition from the beginning of sexual life, while secondary vaginismus occurs sometime after a period of normal sexual function. Vaginismus can be situational when it occurs only on certain circumstances or with certain partners, or global when it occurs regardless of circumstances and partners.

Vaginismus generally presents to doctors with non-consummation of marriage, dyspareunia or difficult gynecologic examination.

What Conditions may Cause Dyspareunia?

Causes of dyspareunia include:

(i) Superficial Dyspareunia

- Lack of vaginal lubrication — poor sexual arousal;
- Chemical irritation from spermicide and/or latex from condom
- Atrophic vaginitis
- Vulvovaginal candidiasis or bacterial vaginosis
- Genital herpes
- Bartholin or Skene gland abscess
- Provoked localized vestibulo-vulvodynia
- Lichen planus
- Lichen sclerosus
- Microfissures on the posterior fourchette
- Crohn's disease
- Vulvo-vaginal trauma
- Post-surgical inflammation and/or scarring; episiotomy
- Female sexual mutilation
- Post-irradiation changes
- Congenital vaginal anomaly/atresia

(ii) Deep Dyspareunia
- Pelvic endometriosis
- Pelvic inflammatory disease
- Pelvic adhesions
- Ovarian cyst
- Irritable bowel syndrome

How is Vaginismus Treated?

Being a phenomenon, rather than a single diagnosis, arising from a vastly diverse etiologic background, vaginismus should be carefully evaluated before its treatment could be formulated. A carefully obtained history on the woman's attitude and cultural perception of sexuality, pregnancy and childbirth, and experience of sexual trauma or abuse is mandatory. A sympathetic and re-assuring approach in getting the woman's co-operation for a clinical examination is essential for the detection of any organic disorders or causes of dyspareunia which can be treated in their specific manners.

In the absence of an organic disorder, the treatment of vaginismus depends on the objective of the woman whether she intends to achieve penetrative vaginal intercourse, use of vaginal tampon, or to become pregnant. For those women seeking a pregnancy, assisted reproduction technique such as intravaginal insemination of sperms or *in vitro* fertilization should be explored.

Women intending to achieve penetrative intercourse are best managed in a program comprising of: (i) sex education and counseling to expel misconceptions on genital hygiene, sexual physiology and reproduction; (ii) desensitization behavioral therapy with gradual exposure to vaginal trainers of increasing sizes to address anxiety related phobias; (iii) sensate focus training through a series of structured touching activities to help couples overcome anxiety and increase comfort with physical intimacy; and (iv) pelvic floor physiotherapy with biofeedback. Some women may also benefit from hypnotherapy.

Selected Diseases

1. Provoked Localized Vestibule-Vulvodynia

Vulvodynia is defined by the International Society for the Study of Vulvo-vaginal Diseases as pain in the vulva for more than three months' duration without a clearly identifiable underlying disease or cause. The estimated incidence of vulvodynia ranges between 3% and 7% among women of reproductive life and is more prevalent in women of age before 25-years. The symptom remits spontaneously in approximately 25% of patients.

Vulvodynia is described in the following categories:

- By location: (i) Generalized vulvodynia where pain is experienced from multiple sites of the vulva; and (ii) localized vulvodynia where pain is limited to one site only.
- By triggering factor: (i) Unprovoked vulvodynia where pain occurs spontaneously; (ii) provoked vulvodynia where pain is elicited by contact, physical exercises, or sexual intercourse; or (iii) mixed type.
- By onset: (i) Primary vulvodynia where the pain is experienced on the first attempt of sexual contact or vaginal tampon insertion; and (ii) secondary vulvodynia where pain develops sometime after painless vulvar contact previously.

The patient presents to doctors with dyspareunic vaginismus, vulvar pain or burning sensation. On clinical examination, the vulva and vestibule are normal except for occasional mild erythema around the openings of the Bartholin glands or Skene glands. There are trigger points on the vestibule upon which pressure provokes an intense pain.

The etiology of the condition is unclear. The affected area is typically free from currently known microbiological agents and the excised tissue exhibits little local inflammatory response. Investigations of the local neuropathways and aberrations in mucosal nerve factors, thermoreceptors and nociceptors have been inconclusive.

The diagnosis of vulvodynia is based on clinical symptoms and by exclusion of known causes of vulvar pain, which include:

- Infective inflammation: e.g. candidiasis, herpes infection
- Non-infective inflammatory conditions: e.g. lichen sclerosus, lichen planus

- Neoplasm: VIN, Paget's disease, vulvar cancer
- Neuralgia: e.g. post-shingle neuralgia, nerve compression, neuroma
- Trauma
- Post-irradiation or local surgery
- Estrogen deficiency.

The aim of treatment is to reduce the pain level and to improve sexual function and psychological well-being of the patient. As the condition appears to be heterogeneous, treatment is individualized and may involve multiple disciplines. Interventional treatment is superior to no-treatment in symptom control. Individual patients may undertake several treatment regimens to achieve clinical benefits.

Treatment regimens for vulvodynia include:

(i) Oral pain control agents
   - Tricyclic antidepressants: amitriptyline
   - Anticonvulsants: gabapentin, pregabalin
   - SSNRIs: duloxetinevenlafaxine

(ii) Topical pain control agents
   - Topical steroid creams
   - Local anesthetic injection

(iii) Local nerve blocks
(iv) Pelvic floor muscle therapy
(v) Psychotherapy
(vi) Surgery:
   - Vestibulectomy where involved vestibule or entire vestibule is excised and the lower vaginal is advanced for wound closure.
   - Modified vestibulectomy where the superficial layer of the involved vestibule is excised without vaginal advancement procedure.
   - Reported success rate of surgery varies according to patient selection.

2. Atrophic Vaginitis

Consequence to estrogen deficiency of menopause, the vagina undergoes a series of changes progressively. Vaginal lubrication diminishes, the expansibility is reduced from loss of mucosal rugae and atrophy of elastic and collagen fibers and the epithelium becomes very thin. This state of degenerative changes is customarily referred to as atrophic vaginitis and the woman experiences varying degree of superficial dyspareunia. The condition, to a large extent, is reversible with estrogen replacement therapy.

Illustration of Some Conditions that Cause Dyspareunia

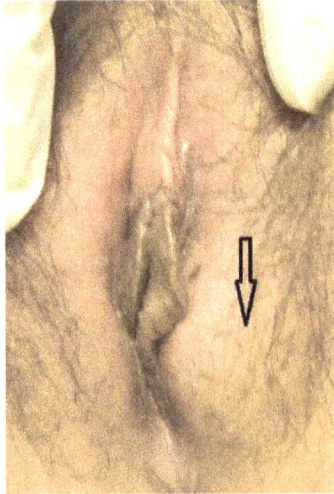

This young woman complained of secondary dyspareunia. The photograph shows a left-sided Bartholin cyst (marked by arrow) without abscess formation.

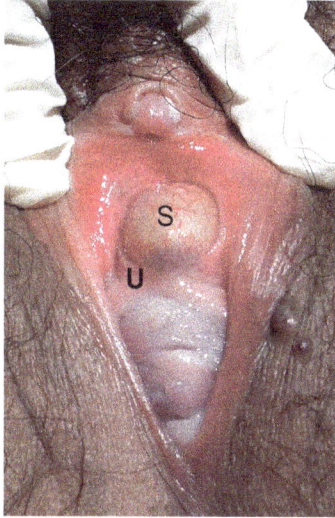

This middle-aged woman had a retention cyst (marked "S") in the Skene gland on the left-hand side. The urethral meatus is marked "U" in this photograph.

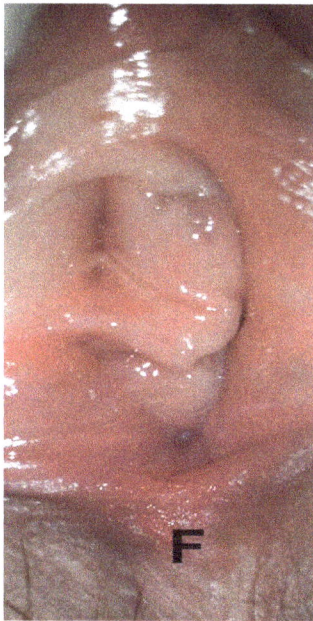

This photograph shows the shadow mucosal break in the posterior fourchette of the vulva (marked "F"). This condition caused superficial dyspareunia.

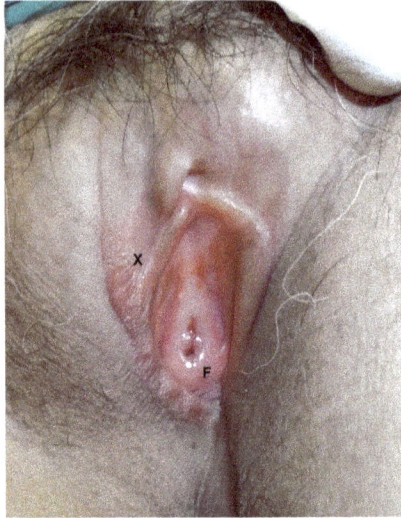

This photograph shows vulva skin afflicted by lichen sclerosus. The labial minora on the right-hand side (marked "X") shows a diminished thickness and the surrounding skin was thin and wrinkling. The overall retraction in the introitus volume causes dyspareunia.

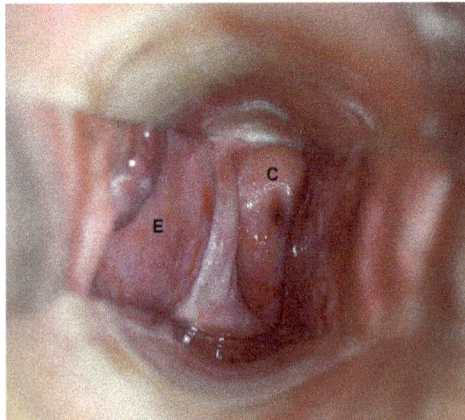

This photograph of a speculum examination shows changes of menopausal atrophic vaginitis. The vagina mucosa was pale and had loss of mucosal rugae.

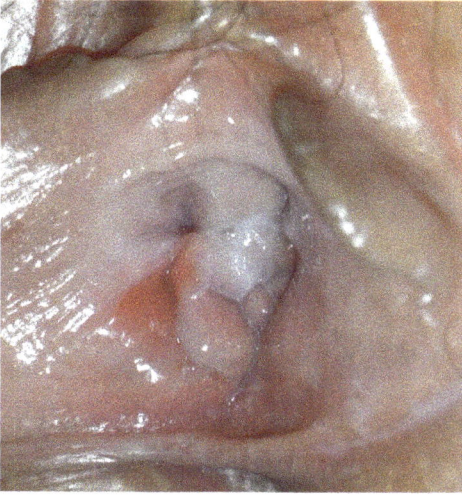

This young woman experienced excruciating dyspareunia. The only positive physical finding was a small area of erythema at the introitus. Gentle pressure applied to this area elicited severe pain identical to dyspareunia. She had vulvodynia.

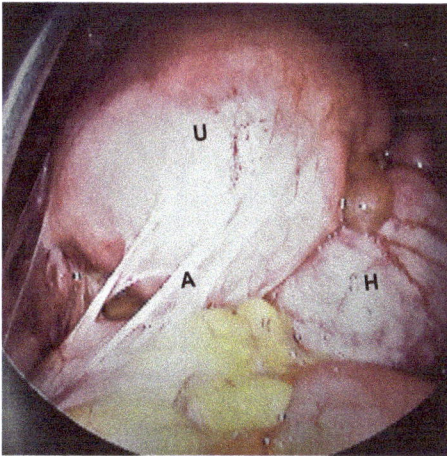

This 35-year-old woman complained of dyspareunia for three months. A diagnostic laparoscopy revealed severe pelvic adhesions from pelvic inflammatory disease.

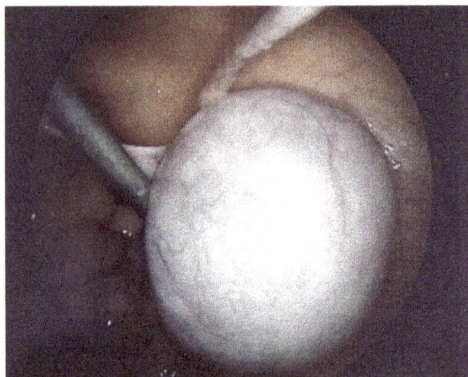

This photograph shows a large ovarian cyst on a laparoscopy. She had a recent history of dyspareunia.

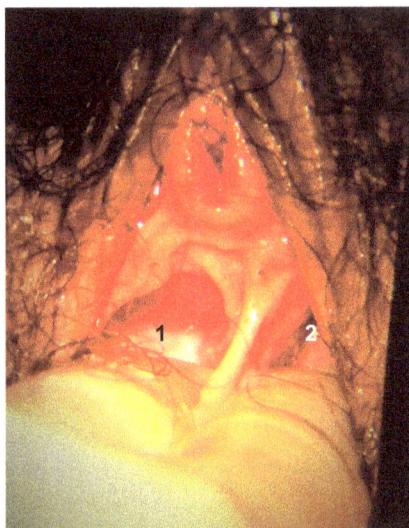

This woman complained of primary dyspareunia. She was found to have a congenital malformation of the genital tract, including double vaginas as demonstrated by two fingers (marked "1" and "2" in the photograph) separated by a fibro-muscular septum.

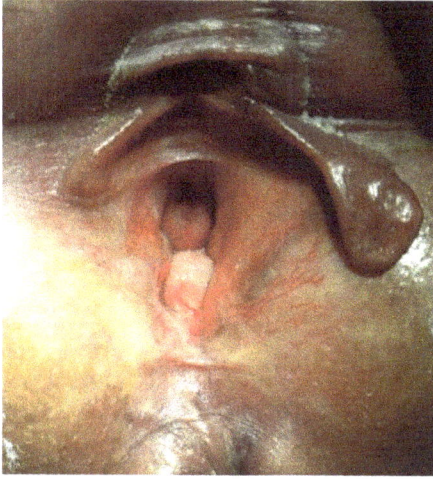

This woman had radiation to the vagina. There is marked post-radiation cutaneous and mucosal atrophy with telangiectasia.

CASE 11 — PREMENSTRUAL SYNDROME

A 20-year-old woman complained of mood swings, irritability and abdominal bloating prior to menstruation.

- What is premenstrual syndrome (PMS)?
- What are the symptoms of PMS and how is the diagnosis established?
- How is PMS managed?

What is Premenstrual Syndrome (PMS)?

Premenstrual syndrome (PMS) describes a set of emotional, physical and behavioral symptoms interfering with the normal activity of the woman during the two weeks prior to onset of menstruation. When the symptoms are extremely severe and morbid, the condition is known as a separate clinical entity of premenstrual dystrophic disorder (PMDD).

The prevalence of PMS in the literature remained similar in the last two decades and was reported in 35% in Africa, 40% in Europe, 45% in Asia and 60% in South America. A wide variation in the prevalence between different studies was likely a reflection of the sample size of the studies. It is estimated that nearly 20% of women are affected by clinically significant PMS and 3% are PMDD. The prevalence of moderate to severe symptoms of PMS is most common in older adolescents and young women, but the condition often persists or recurs later and resolves only upon menopause.

Recent studies do not support a long-held belief that PMS is caused by a dysfunctional pituitary-ovarian axis with imbalance in the ratio of estrogen-progesterone levels. The current consensus holds the view that, in PMS, the normal ovarian function repeatedly triggers a serotonin-related biochemical events in the central nervous system. Other postulated theories of PMS include psycho-social conflicts between femininity and motherhood, cognitive and maladaptation of stress coping mechanism for menstruation and premenstrual symptoms, and sociocultural conflicts between economic productivity and child-bearing roles of the woman.

What are the Symptoms of PMS and How is the Diagnosis Established?

For the diagnosis of PMS or PMDD, the symptoms must occur within the luteal phase of the menstrual cycle and resolve soon after the onset of menstruation. PMS must be differentiated from premenstrual exacerbation of a pre-existing affective or physical disorder. Secondly, the symptoms must be of sufficient severity to interfere with the woman's daily function.

Diagnosis of PMS is based on changes of symptoms between the follicular and luteal phases over at least two consecutive menstrual cycles. Physical examination and laboratory investigations do not contribute positively to the diagnosis but may be informative in establishing other disorders with symptoms mimicking PMS, such as thyroid disorder.

The symptoms of PMS include:

(i) **Psycho-emotional Symptoms**
- Depressed or labile mood
- Anxiety
- Irritability
- Anger

(ii) **Behavioral Symptoms**
- Decreased interest in daily activities
- Difficulty in concentrating
- Change in appetite, overeating, or specific food cravings
- Sleep disturbance — hypersomnia or insomnia
- A subjective sense of being overwhelmed or out of control

(iii) **Physical Symptoms**
- Lethargy and easy fatigability
- Breast tenderness or swelling
- Sensation of bloating or weight gain
- Headaches
- Joint or muscle pain.

How is PMS Managed?

The patient must be educated that treatment of PMS is a long process and the symptoms cannot be completely eradicated by any single therapy. A combination of the following approach may be needed either simultaneously or at different stages of the evolution of the condition.

(i) Non-pharmacology Treatments

Therapy. Acupuncture and bright light therapy are associated with symptomatic improvement in depression for PMS. Sleep deprivation therapy has reported improvement in depression after the night of recovery sleep. Cognitive-behavioral therapy to replace negative thoughts and feelings with positive and adaptive views has also been reported to be effective in managing anger and negative emotions.

Dietary modification constitutes an important component of non-pharmacological treatment of PMS:

- Reducing caffeine intake to minimize the potential adverse effects of excess caffeine consumption (e.g. nervousness, jitteriness).
- Restricting sodium intake may reduce bloating.
- Replacing intake of highly refined carbohydrates which contain complex carbohydrates and by having five or six smaller meals during the day instead of three large meals in the late luteal phase to improve mood, appetite, and cognitive function.

Nutritional supplements

- Vitamin B complex
- Calcium with magnesium chloride
- Evening primrose oil
- *L*-tyrosine
- Multivitamin-mineral complex with manganese
- Vitamin C with bioflavonoids

Exercise. Moderate aerobic exercise improved premenstrual symptoms, particularly if depressive or fluid retention symptoms predominate.

(ii) Pharmacologic Treatment of PMS

Pharmocological treatment aims to reduce the severity of the symptoms. Daily Record of Severity of Problems Scores in PMDD has been shown to show greater improvement with combined drospirenone-ethinyl estradiol pills than placebo. Improvement in premenstrual symptoms has also been reported with the use of estrogen, progestogen, combined oral contraceptive pills, danazol and GnRH analogues. The choice of these agents depends on the profile of adverse effects of the individual agent. Spironolactone and other diuretics are used widely to treat many symptoms of PMS secondary to fluid retention. Nonsteroidal anti-inflammatory drugs (NSAIDs), including mefanamic acid, naprosen and COX-2 inhibitors yielded greater improvement of premenstrual symptoms than placebo. However, it is selective serotonin reuptake inhibitors (SSRIs) such as fluoxetine, sertraline, and controlled-release paroxetine that are emerging as the most effective treatment option for severe symptoms of PMS and PMDD. A Cochrane review reported that all SSRIs have excellent efficacy and minimal adverse effects. The used of SSRIs in young adolescent, however, is not recommended.

CASE 12 — VAGINAL DISCHARGE

A 26-year-old woman complains of excessive vaginal discharge for two weeks.

- What is the origin of physiological vaginal discharge and how is it distinguished from pathological discharge?
- What conditions may manifest by vaginal discharge?
- When and what laboratory investigations are indicated for vaginal discharge?

What is the Origin of Physiological Vaginal Discharge and How is it Distinguished from Pathological Discharge?

Normal vaginal fluid is made up of serous or watery vaginal transudate and secretions from the fallopian tubes and peritoneum, and mucus secretion from the cervix and uterus. Estrogen and progesterone exert a profound effect on the physical property of cervical secretion which manifest in changes in the characteristics and volume of vaginal fluid observed throughout a menstrual cycle. In the follicular phase, vaginal fluid is watery and transparent and the volume increases towards ovulatory period with rising estrogen level. In the luteal phase, the predominant progesterone influence increases the viscosity of the cervical secretion and the vaginal fluid becomes scanty, thick and opaque, producing the ferning and spinbarkeit phenomenon. The hormone-dependent physiological variation in vaginal fluid is diminished in women on combined oral contraceptive pills. The vaginal secretion becomes very scanty in amount and viscous in consistency in women on progestogen-only contraceptives.

There is a marked variation in the volume of vaginal secretion between individuals. The amount of discharge is also influenced by the volume of seminal fluid of recent sexual intercourse. Examining doctor must bear in mind that a mere discovery of copious discharge during vaginal examination does not necessarily indicate an on-going pathology. Pathological vaginal discharge is suspected by the woman's own observation of a deviation in the characteristics and amount of vaginal secretion from her normal experience. The probability of a discharge being pathological increases when other features are present, such as discoloration in the discharge, presence of an odor and/or vulvo-vaginal itch, blood staining in the discharge, post-coital bleeding, and recent onset of dyspareunia.

What Conditions may Manifest by Vaginal Discharge?

The pathological causes of vaginal discharge include:

(i) *Vaginal Infection*
  • Bacterial vaginosis
  • Vaginal candidiasis
  • Sexually transmitted infections (STI), such as Trichomoniasis, Gonorrhea and Chlamydia
  • Post-gynecological surgical infection
(ii) *Retained Foreign Body* — tampon, condom, or vaginal sponge.
(iii) *Inflammation* due to allergy or irritation caused by deodorants, lubricants, and disinfectants.
(iv) *Atrophic Vaginitis* in post-menopausal women.
(v) Cervical ectropion or polyps.
(vi) *Tumors* of the vulva, vagina, cervix, and endometrium.
(vii) *Urinary Incontinence*
(viii) *Vesico-vaginal or Rectovaginal fistulae.*

When and What Laboratory Investigations are Indicated for Vaginal Discharge?

It is accepted that not all cases of vaginal discharge require laboratory investigation before initiation of treatment, particularly for the following group of women:

- Women below 25-years old
- Women assessed to be at low risk of STIs
- Vaginal discharge has the characteristics of candidiasis, bacterial vaginosis or trichomoniasis.

(i) Laboratory Investigations are Indicated for these Women

- Assessed to be at high risk of an STI
- Cervicitis seen on examination
- Suspected PID
- A poor response to initial treatment, or recurrent vaginal discharge
- Discharge of uncertain cause
- Discharge after a gynecological procedure or childbirth.

(ii) Laboratory Investigations to be Considered

Samples for laboratory tests include a high vaginal swab (HVS) of discharge taken from the lateral vaginal wall and posterior fornix, and endocervical swab (ECS) taken from the endocervix, after cleaning the cervical os with a large sterile swab.

- VP3 — This is a rapid and automated DNA-based test on HVS for detection of candida, bacterial vaginosis and trichomoniasis. The sensitivity and specificity are 80% and 95%, respectively for candida (included species *C. albicans*, *C. glabrata*, *C. kefyr*, *C. krusei*, *C. parapsilosis*, and *C. tropicalis*), 90% and 98%, respectively for *Gardnerella vaginalis,* and 93% and 90%, respectively for *Trichomonas vaginalis.*

- PCR tests for chlamydia and gonorrhoea — Qualitative PCR-based tests using either a probe targeting DNA sequence or RNA sequence of *Chlamydia trachomatis* and *Neisseria gonorrhea* are available. The reported sensitivity and specificity of the test for *Chlamydia trachomatis* and *N. gonorrhea* in ECS are above 90% and 99%, respectively.
- Microbiological culture and antibiotic sensitivity tests for gonorrhea and other bacteria — this is an important investigation in the diagnosis of bacterial infection and antibiotic sensitivity test.

Selected Diseases

1. Vulvo-vaginal Candidiasis

During the reproductive life of a woman, the vagina maintains a moist environment with a pH value fluctuating between 3.8 and 4.5, maintained by the lactic acid produced by the actions of *Lactobacillus and Corynebacterium* on vaginal epithelial glycogen. The acidic milieu renders other vaginal aerobic and anaerobic gram-positive and gram-negative bacteria non-pathogenic. These bacteria include Streptococcus, Bacteroides, Staphylococcus, and Peptostreptococcus. Approximately 50% of women are also opportunistic carriers of Candida albicans.

Vulvo-vaginal candidiasis is an inflammatory condition of the vagina, vulva and the adjacent crural areas caused by candida, most commonly by C. albicans (90%) and less commonly by C. glabrata, C. tropicalis and C. krusei. It occurs most commonly during the childbearing age and a woman's life-time risk is 75% for at least one episode of vulvo-vaginal candidiasis. It is not considered a sexually transmitted disease.

The risk factors for vulvo-vaginal candidiasis include:

- Pregnancy: the high estrogen state of pregnancy lowers the vaginal pH which suppresses other vaginal microbial flora and promotes overgrowth of candida. It is estimated that, at any day, a third of pregnant woman are affected by vulvo-vaginal candidiasis.

- Combined oral contraceptive pills: high-dose estrogen containing contraceptives pills were associated with a high prevalence of vulvo-vaginal candidiasis for the same reason as pregnancy. The new generations of low-dose contraceptive pills have not been found to increase the users' risk of vulvo-vaginal candidiasis.
- Antibiotics: use of broad spectrum antibiotics, by killing the other vaginal microbials, facilitates overgrowth of candida and the development of clinical vulvo-vaginal candidiasis.
- Immunosuppression: HIV infection, auto-immune disorders, immunosuppresants are associated with a high prevalence of candidiasis.

Acute vulvo-vaginal candidiasis presents with an intense itch and burning sensation in the vulva and the adjacent areas. There may be accompanied by dyspareunia. Erythema and edema may be seen at the vestibule, labia majora and minora and the rash may extend to the thighs and perineum. The vaginal discharge is typically white or light yellow in color and thick or curd-like in consistency, sometimes forming thrush patches on the vaginal wall and vulva.

Acute vulvo-vaginal candidiasis with typical clinical presentation in a woman at low risk of sexually transmitted disease does not require laboratory investigations. The clinical and mycotic cure rate with the azole group of anti-mycotic agents is 90%.

2. Bacterial Vaginosis (BV)

BV is one of the most common reasons for women seeking treatment for vaginal discharge. It affects 20% to 25% of pregnant women and 40% of women attending sexual health clinics. It has a characteristic white or greyish homogenous vaginal discharge with a pH of 4.5 or greater. The discharge may carry a fishing odor, which is the most prevalent after sexual intercourse as the alkaline seminal fluid reacts with the discharge to release volatile amines.

BV can occur and regress spontaneously. Although commonly found in sexually active women, it is not considered a sexually transmitted disease. Instead, there is an overgrowth of anaerobic bacteria in place of lactobacilli. The most commonly associated bacteria in BV is *Gardnerella vaginalis*. Other involved bacteria include *Prevotella* species, *Mycoplasma hominis* and *Mobiluncus* species.

Risk factors for BV include recent use of antibiotics, decrease estrogen level, use of intrauterine contraceptive device and vaginal douching.

Physical examination shows a pool of thin discharge with small bubbles in the posterior vaginal fornix. Typically, there is no associated cervical, vaginal or vulvar inflammation. Clinical diagnosis of BV can be confirmed on microscopic examination of the discharge by the presence of clue cells (epithelial cells studded with bacteria on the surface) and absence of polymorphs, and a positive KOH test (release of amines by adding a drop of 10% KOH to a drop of vaginal discharge on a microscopic slide). Microbiologic culture is indicated only in cases suspicious of or in women at high risk of sexually transmitted diseases.

Treatment of BV includes stopping usage of vaginal douching and strong body soap. Medical treatment is indicated for pregnant women, women on IUCD and before gynecological surgery. Metronidazole is the most commonly used medical treatment of BV. The cure rate is more than 80%. Clindamicin, a more expensive medication than metronidazole, carries a comparable effectiveness as metronidazole. Treatment of male partner is not necessary as it is not associated with a higher cure rate or prevention of recurrence of BV.

3. Trichomoniasis Vaginalis (T. vaginalis)

In women, trichomoniasis is a parasitic infection of vaginal, urethra, and Skene and Bartholin glands by flagellated trichomonad protozoa. This is one of the most commonly diagnosed STIs, with an estimated prevalence of 170 million cases worldwide. The prevalence increases with age, from 2.3% among adolescents aged 18–24 years to 4% among adults 25 years and older, and an overall prevalence of 3.1% in females aged 14–49 years.

Almost 80% of women with vaginal trichomoniasis are asymptomatic. In symptomatic cases, the most common presentations are vaginal discharge with a musty odor, vulvo-vaginal itching and soreness, dyspareunia and post-coital bleeding, and dysuria. Physical examination reveals cervicitis with muco-purulent endocervical discharge and contact bleeding. When present, the strawberry or patchy erythematous appearance of the cervix (colpitis macularis) is pathognomonic of trichomoniasis vaginalis.

Untreated cases of trichomoniasis vaginalis may cause inflammatory disease of the Bartholin glands and Skene glands, endometritis and salpingo-oophoritis or abscess. Vaginal trichomoniasis is associated with an increased risk of HIV infection and development of cervical intraepithelial neoplasia. Infection during pregnancy may also be complicated by preterm labor.

Diagnosis of *T. vaginalis* is based on laboratory tests. Microscopy detection of flagellated oval trichomonads amid plethora polymorph is diagnostic of *T. vaginitis*. The test, however, carries a low sensitivity of about 70%. DNA probe-based test is now available for rapid detection of this infection and has largely replaced laboratory culture test. Microbiological culture tests and serological screening for HIV and hepatitis for concomitant STIs are essential in providing a comprehensive care of these women.

Prompt treatment of *T. vaginalis* is indicated. The standard treatment is metronidazole 2 g orally as a single dose, including during pregnancy. Treatment of asymptomatic pregnant women may be delayed until 37 weeks gestation.

Illustration of Some Conditions that Cause Vaginal Discharge

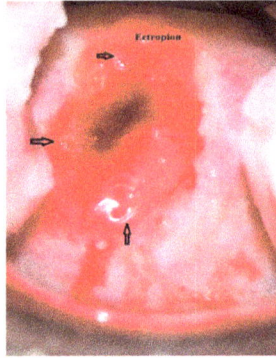

This photograph shows the cervix of a young woman. A layer of transparent secretion (marked by arrows) covers the area of cervical ectropion. This cervico-vaginal secretion is physiological, found in the luteal and peri-ovulatory phases of the menstrual cycle.

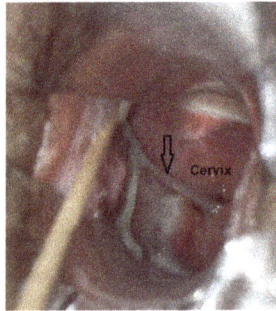

This photograph shows strains (marked by the arrow) of thick and stretchy mucoid discharge from the cervix in a woman in the luteal phase of the menstrual cycle.

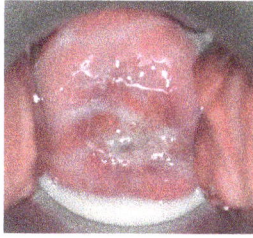

This photograph shows copious watery discharge in a young woman. There was no cervicitis or vulvo-vaginitis. The discharge was not pathological.

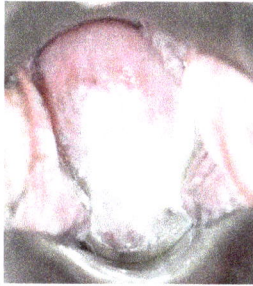

This 29-year-old woman on long-tern combined estrogen-progestagen contraceptive pills was found to have abundant thick vaginal discharge covering the cevix. She was asymptomatic and examination of the lower genital tract did not reveal any vulvo-vaginal inflammatory changes. The discharge is physiological.

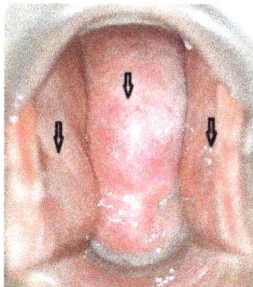

This 70-year-old woman had atrophic vaginitis with a small pool of thick yellowish discharge in the posterior vaginal fornix. The vagina mucosa (marked by arrows) was smooth and thin. The condition resolved on topical vaginal estrogen treatment.

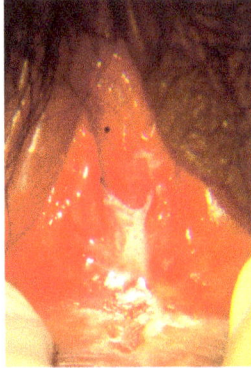

This photograph illustrates excessive yellowish vaginal diacharge seen at the introitus of the vagina from acute candidiasis. There was associated swelling at the vulva minora.

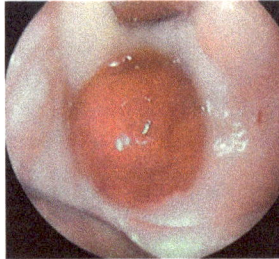

Cervical polyp, as shown in this photograph, often presents with abnormal vaginal bleeding. In some cases, the patient may complain of a vaginal discharge.

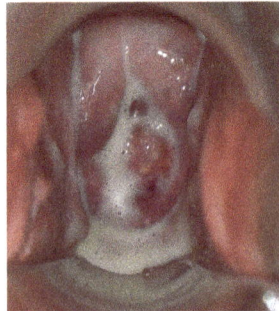

This photograph shows copious greyish frothy discharge in a young woman with bacterial vaginosis.

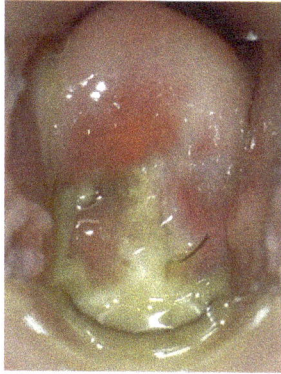

This photograph illustrates a woman in whom the dischage was caused by cervicitis associated with intrauterine contraceptive device (the arrow points to the string of the device).

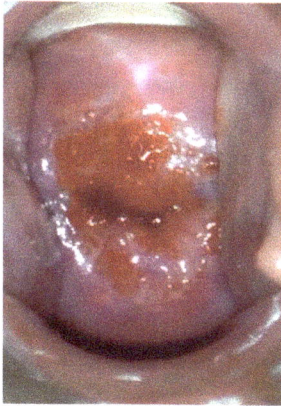

This 25-year-old woman complained of recent onset of increased vaginal discharge and post-coital bleeding. After vaginal discharge was cleared during examination, the cervix was found to be acutely inflamed.

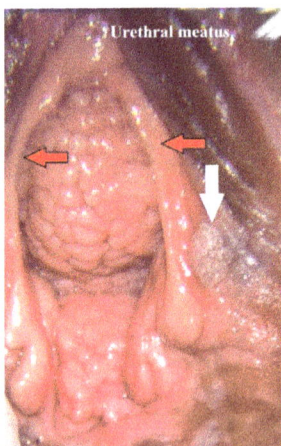

This 32-year-old woman complained of a vaginal discharge. She had a genital wart (*Condyloma acuminata*) at the vestibule (white arrow). The remnants of the hymen are indicated by red arrows on this photograph.

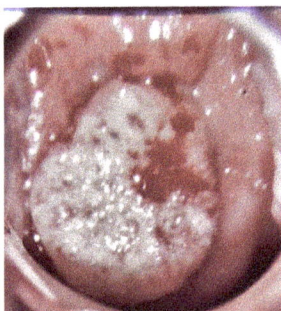

This 60-year-old woman who complained of increasing vaginal discharge was found to have carcinoma of the cervix. The tumor showed inflammatory exudate on the surface as shown in this photograph.

CASE 13 — PRURITUS VULVAE

A 60-year-old woman complains of a persistent itch on the vulva.

- What history in the symptom is helpful in understanding the etiology of pruritus vulvae?
- What are the common conditions that cause pruritus vulvae?

What History in the Symptom is Helpful in Understanding the Etiology of Pruritus Vulvae?

A persistent itch or pruritus is an unpleasant sensation that provokes a desire to scratch. A number of substances are known to induce itch via stimulation of nociceptive neurons superficially located in the epidermis and subepidermal tissues. These include inflammatory mediators such as histamine, neuropeptide substance P, serotonin, bradykinin, tryptase from mast cells, and endothelin. Other substances that have been postulated to cause an itch in systemic diseases, such as urea from chronic renal failure, bile salts from cholestasis or primary biliary cirrhosis, iron from hematological disorders, parathyroid hormone and thyroid hormones have thus far found little supporting evidence.

Pruritus vulvae is a pruritic condition limited to the vulvo-vagino-perineal region. Vulva and perineal skin, including the non-hair bearing part of the vaginal introitus shares the same structure as the rest of the body skin and are exposed to the same etiological factors and causes of itch. These include dermatological disorders, local inflammation or infection, chronic systemic diseases and malignancy. The upper part of the vaginal, like the rest of the internal organs, does not bear itch receptors and does not manifest an itch sensation.

Attention is needed in taking a reliable history to make a clear distinction of pruritus from vulva pain or burning sensation. The first attention is to determine if the itch is associated with a change in vaginal discharge as it indicates a vulvo-vaginitis etiology (see "vaginal discharge"). A diagnosis of vulvo-vaginitis can be reached with the typical quantitative and/or qualitative changes in vaginal discharge.

In the absence of vaginal discharges, a history of recurrent itch and rash on the vulva and other parts of the body is a strong indicator of some dermatological disorders, such as eczema and psoriasis. However, acute vulvo-vaginitis can add to the symptoms of chronic dermatoses.

What are the Common Conditions that Cause Pruritus Vulvae?

The common causes of pruritus vulvae can be classified by history of the symptoms into acute and chronic categories.

(A) Causes of Acute Pruritus Vulvae

(i) Allergic or Irritant Contact Dermatitis
   a. Hygiene products such as skin wipes, antiseptics, scented toilet paper and sanitary pads, and soaps and shampoos
   b. Condoms, vaginal contraceptives and lubricants
   c. Topical medications such as anesthetics, antibacterials, trichloroacetic acid, 5-fluorouracil, podophyllin and imiqui-mod cream.

(ii) Vulvo-vaginal Infections
   a. Fungal infections (candidiasis and tinea cruris)
   b. Bacterial vaginosis
   c. Trichomoniasis

  d. Scabies
  e. Molluscum contagiosum
  f. Genital warts

(B) Causes of Chronic Pruritus Vulvae

(i) Dermatoses
  a. Atopic and contact dermatitis
  b. Psoriasis
  c. Lichen sclerosus
  d. Lichen planus
  e. Lichen simplex chronicus

(ii) Neoplastic Lesions
  a. Vulvar intraepithelial neoplasia
  b. Vulvar cancer
  c. Paget's disease

(C) Crohn's Disease: Vulvar Manifestation of Systemic Disease

Selected Diseases

1. Vulvar Lichen Sclerosus (VLS)

Lichen sclerosus is a chronic inflammatory skin condition with characteristic histological changes: the epidermis shows hyperkeratosis, thinning of the malphigian layer, flattening or absence of pete ridges; and the dermis shows edema with loss of elastic fibers in the upper dermis, and aggregation of inflammatory infiltrates in the lower dermis. Lichen sclerosus can affect both men and women of any age, but is more prevalent in the two extremes of life in women. In women, lichen sclerosus is most prevalent in the vulva. It has been variously estimated to affect 1 in 70 to 1 in 1000 women, and is said to be more common in Caucasians than in Asian women.

VLS is believed to be an autoimmune disorder, being more common in some families and being frequently associated with other autoimmune phenomena such as thyroid disorders, diabetes mellitus, anemia, vitiligo and alopecia areata.

Clinical presentations of VLS appear in phases.

(i) **Pruritus vulvae.** The affected skin is chronically itchy, the intensity of which varies and tends to be worse at night and may cause severe sleep disturbance. The affected skin appears as paper thin, white or silvery patches with surface wrinkling.

(ii) **Vulvar pain.** Scratches produce skin traumas and fissures which are painful.

(iii) **Dyspareunia.** Painful sexual intercourse may arise from fissures or vulvo-vaginal contractures. VLS typically causes atrophy or loss of labia minora and formation of synechiae which may cause the labia to fuse together or obscure the clitoris. In long-standing cases, tissue distortions result in constriction of the introitus previously termed kraurosis.

(iv) **Malignancy.** Among squamous cell carcinoma of the vulva, particularly among the older women, 50% are not associated with human papillomavirus infection and are known to have an associated VLS. The progression of VLS to cancer has been estimated to be approximately 5%.

Management of VLS involves a vulva biopsy for a definitive diagnosis. Repeated biopsies may be needed for long-term surveillance of the disease progression and early detection of malignancy. Patients should be counselled that VLS is a lifelong disorder and the aim of management is to alleviate symptoms and reduce progression of the disease. The mainstay treatment is daily topical application of a strong steroid (clobetasol proprionate) oilment for 3–4 months and a long-term maintenance steroid cream treatment. Surgical treatment is reserved for correction of sequelae of VLS such as labial fusion and synechiae.

2. Vulvar Intraepithelial Neoplasia (VIN)

VIN, a pre-malignant lesion on the vulva, is categorized into two distinct subtypes: (a) HPV-16 associated VIN known as the usual-type VIN (uVIN); and (b) differentiated type (dVIN) independent of HPV.

uVIN occurs in younger women and appears as multifocal raised plagues; some are pigmented. They are usually identified on colposcopy during evaluation of cervical neoplasia and are treated at the same time. Consequently, progression of uVIN to squamous cell carcinoma of the vulva is uncommon and has been estimated to be about 5%. This risk is higher among immunosuppressed women above 35-years-old.

dVIN occurs in postmenopausal women with a mean age of 68-years. It appears as an ill-defined unifocal white or red plague, often associated with a chronic condition such as VLS. In more than 60% of cases, dVIN is pruritic. dVIN is a high-grade lesion with a potential to progress to invasive squamous cell carcinoma in 30% of untreated cases.

Management of both uVIN and dVIN is the same. In unifocal lesion, local excision confers an excellent primary cure rate. In multifocal uVIN or coalescent uVIN, which are more common among young women with low risk of invasive cancer, laser vaporization therapy is an appropriate and efficient treatment. Medical treatment of VIN with imiquimod cream is a promising alternative treatment to surgical treatment.

3. Vulvar Paget's Disease (also known as Extra-mammary Paget's Disease)

Paget's disease of the vulva presents as single or multiple red lesions on the vulva. It is often itchy and may become eczematous and painful at time. The diagnosis is based on histology which shows typical groups of clear-looking tumor cells scattered among keratocytes of the epidermis. These cells show characteristic immunohistochemical property, i.e. staining positive for cytokeratin-7 and negative for melanin. The finding of these lesions almost exclusively in skin rich, apocrine glands gives rise to the theory that the cells have an origin from the apocrine cells. An alternative hypothesis suggests that these neoplastic cells are migratory in origin as Paget's disease is commonly associated with gastrointestinal tract malignancy. It is important to investigate all patients with Paget's disease of the vulva for malignancies in skin appendages or gastrointestinal tract. Also of great clinical significance is to note that more than 50% of untreated Paget's disease of the vulva progress to invasive carcinoma.

The mainstay treatment of Paget's disease of the vulva is surgical excision. Because of the migratory nature of these tumor cells, the completeness of excision is difficult to achieve without an extensive procedure. Long-term surveillance is required for early detection of disease relapses, either in the grafted tissues or in the tissue adjacent to excision, and for potential development of malignancy.

There is emerging evidence that some lesions of the Paget's disease may respond to topical application of imiquimod cream. The long-term outcome of this form of treatment is yet lacking.

4. Vulvar Cancer

Vulvar cancer is similar to skin cancer elsewhere on the body, with the great majority being squamous cell carcinoma. Less commonly, there are adenocarcinoma and melanoma. Vulvar cancer accounts for 5% of all gynecological cancers and is predominantly a disease of the elderly; 70% of the patients are above 60-years old and 15% are above 80 years old. In Singapore, the proportion of cases above 60-years old seems to be increasing over the last 40 years.

The main symptoms of vulvar cancer are: itch or burning sensation or pain at the site of the lesion. The lesion may show skin discoloration (white, red, brown to black) and may appear as a lump or an ulcer. More than 75% of vulvar cancers are found in the labia. There may be palpable groin lymphadenopathy from tumor metastasis.

Vulvar cancer is classified by the FIGO into four stages, according to tumor dimension, depth of stromal invasion, lymphatic metastasis and involvement of the adjacent or distant viscera or organs.

Stage-I. Tumor ≤2 cm and confined to the labia or perineum, and no lymphatic metastasis. Stage-IA is a tumor invading ≤0.5 mm into the stroma and stage-IB is tumor invading the stroma for more than 0.5 mm but less than 1 mm.

Stage-II. Tumor as in stage-1 but the depth of invasion into stroma exceeds 1 mm.

Stage-III. Tumor of any size with lymph node metastasis limited to the groin. Stage-IIIA for one lymph node of 5 mm or greater in dimension or two lymph nodes of less than 5 mm in diameter. Stage-IIIB refers to metastasis involving two or more lymph nodes ≥5 mm or three or more lymph nodes ≤5 mm in dimensions. Stage-IIIC refers to metastasis extending beyond lymph node capsular tissue.

Stage-IV. Tumor involving other viscera or organs. Stage-IVA refers to tumor involving upper 2/3 of urethra or vagina, or bladder mucosa, rectal mucosa or fixed to pelvic bones. Stage-IVB is defined by any distant metastasis beyond stage-IVA.

The mainstay treatment for vulvar cancer is surgical excision. Stage-1 vulvar cancers can be treated with excellent cure rate with local wide excision alone. Larger tumor should be treated with vulvectomy with groin lymph node dissection. For tumors involving both sides of the vulva or encroaching onto the clitoris, radical vulvectomy with bilateral groin lymphadenectomy is the surgical option of choice. Locally advanced tumors deemed unresectable can be treated with concurrent chemo-radiation.

A good prognosis with a 5-year survival rate of 85% to 90% can be achieved for Stage-1 carcinoma of the vulva. For tumors with lymph node metastasis, the 5-year survival rate is approximately 40%.

Illustration of Some Conditions that Cause Pruritus Vulvae

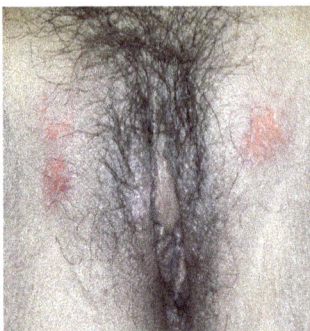

This photograph shows the scratch marks from a case of pruritus vulvae. The excoriated areas become painful. A distinction must be drawn between the primary symptom of pruritus and the secondary symptom of pain.

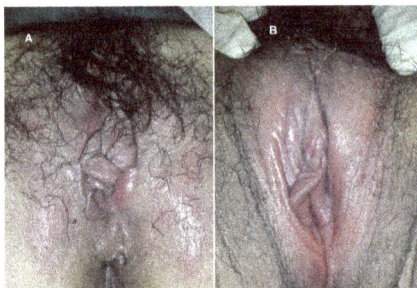

These photographs show the pruritic rashes from contact dermatoses (A) and chronic application of soap washes (B).

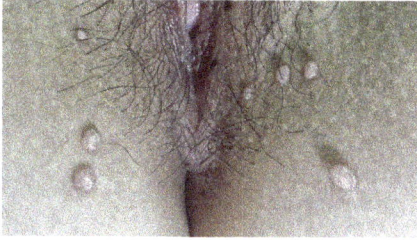

This 30-year-old woman complained of intense itchy lesions on the vulva and inner aspect of the thighs. This photograph shows crops of molluscum contagiosum. The size of the lesions ranges from a pin-head to 5-mm in diameter and, typically, the lesions may be white or pink in color, with a dimple in the center. Molluscum contagiosum is caused by a poxvirus which is highly contagious, and scratching of the lesions will lead to inoculation of the virus to the surrounding skin or elsewhere on the body. The lesions resolved spontaneously without leaving any scars on the skin.

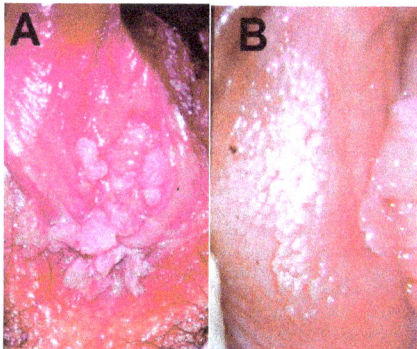

This 28-year-old woman complained of pruritus vulvae 2 weeks after a new sexual contact. A crop of genital warts (condylomata acuminata) is shown in panel (A). Caution is called to make a distinction of small genital warts from a common condition of micropapillary epithelial proliferations in the mucosal aspect of the vulva in young women (panel (B)).

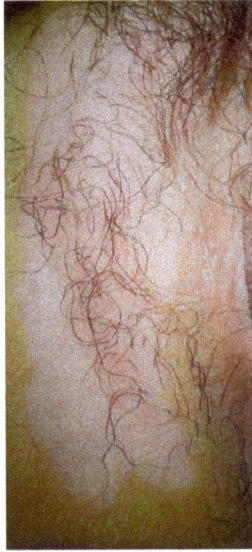

Psoriasis can occur in the vulva alone, although more commonly, vulvar psoriasis is part of the manifestation of a generalized psoriasis. In the vulva, psoriasis involves the labia majora and may extend to the groin areas. The lesion is typically salmon-red and has a well demarcated border. It may be asymptomatic or pruritic intermittently.

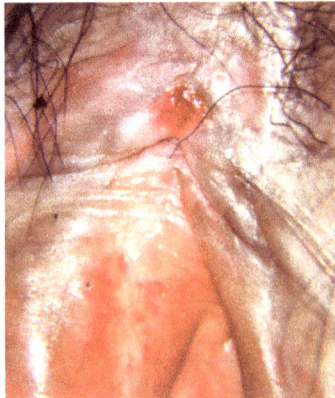

This post-menopausal woman complained of a long standing pruritus vulvae. The atrophy vulva displayed white and thin VLS with scratch traumas.

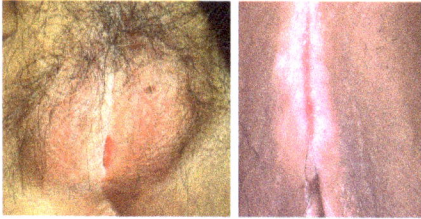

These photographs show two women with severe VLS that distorted the vulvar anatomy. The photograph on the right shows adhesion obscuring the clitoris. The photograph on the left shows that the introitus was reduced to a small orifice.

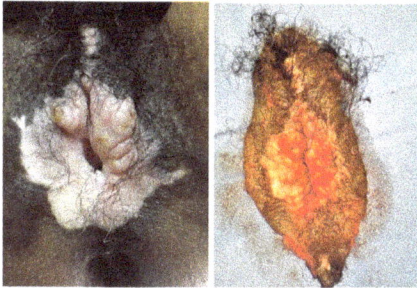

The photographs on the left shows a woman with a large area of VLS (white arrow). There was marked anatomical distortion of the vulva. Tumor developed within the VLS. She undertook a radical vulvectomy as shown in the photographs on the right hand side of the panel.

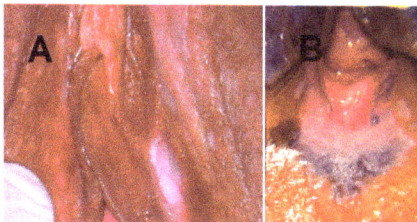

These photographs show uVIN as a unifocal white plague (A), and a diffuse white patch with pigmented areas in (B).

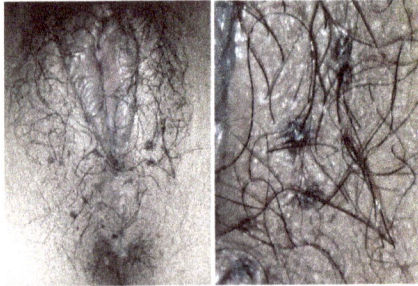

This 35-year-old woman on long-term steroid therapy for chronic systemic lupus erythematosus had multiple black-mole-like lesions over the labia majora and perineum. These lesions were HPV-related undifferentiated VIN.

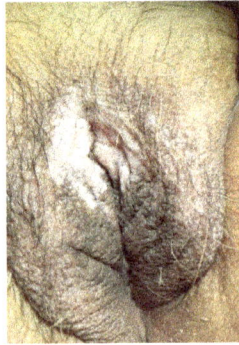

This photograph shows a white patch of dVIN on the vulva of an elderly woman.

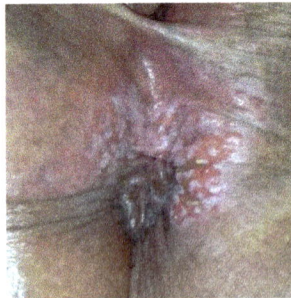

This photograph shows a red patch of Paget's disease on the perineum and perianal area of a woman.

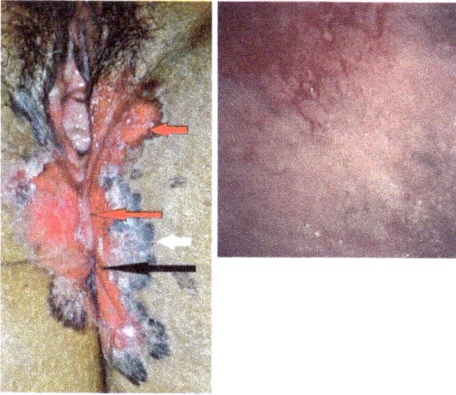

This 39-year-old woman complained of a mild itch at the vulva intermittently. She had undertaken treatment for genital warts 5 years previously. The photographs on the left shows an extensive lesion involving the labia bilaterally, the perineum and the perianal areas. The lesion was red in color with a pigmented periphery. The raised areas at the left labia and perineum (red arrows) were proven to harbor an invasive squamous cell carcinoma. The pigmented periphery (white arrow) was VIN3. The black arrow indicates the anus. The photographs on the right was taken with colposcopy to show the epithelial topography of early invasive squamous cell carcinoma of the vulva. She was positive on HPV-16 DNA test.

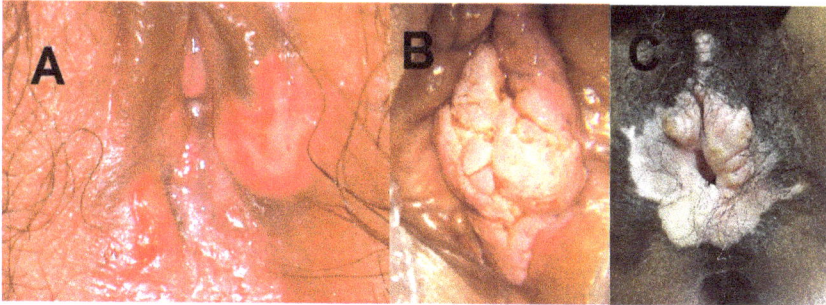

Three cases of vulvar carcinoma are illustrated here: (A) an ulcerated lesion, (B) a large exophytic tumor, and (C) a tumor arising from a long standing lichen sclerosus.

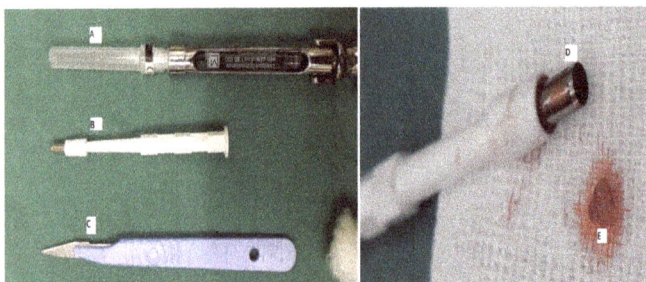

Biopsy of the vulva in a clinic office: (A) Dental syringe with local anesthetic; (B) Keyes skin biopsy device; (C) scalpel; (D) the cutting end of Keyes biopsy device; and (E) a full-thickness biopsy sample of the vulva.

CASE 14 — PAINFUL VULVA

A 29-year-old woman with no prior pregnancy complains of a pain down below.

- What history is important in evaluating the cause of the pain?
- What are the common conditions causing pain in the vulva?

What History is Important in Evaluating the Cause of the Pain?

Pain is a distressing symptom arising from a large variety of causes, sometimes with an obvious lesion but, not infrequently, with no apparent abnormality found at the location of the complaint. A detail history is mandatory and should include the following aspects:

(i) **Nature of Pain.** It is important to determine if the pain is sharp, dull ache or burning in nature, and whether it is an intermittent pain with known aggravating factors or a persistent pain. Pain score is a useful measure for assessing severity of pain and for subsequent monitoring on its response to treatment.

(ii) **History of Pain.** An acute onset of pain is more likely to be caused by a specific condition or a complication superimposed on a chronic vulvar condition. A long-standing or chronic pain may be a manifestation of diseases unrelated to gynecological conditions and should alert the physician to investigate more comprehensively, including the emotional, psychological and psychiatric aspects.

(iii) **Prior Treatment.** The type and response to prior treatment may throw light on the etiology of the pain. Topical treatment for an alleged fungal infection may induce local irritation and pain. Repeated steroidal treatment for an itch may highlight an underlying lichen sclerosus where fissures are painful. Topical treatment for genital warts with podophylin, trichloroacetic acid or imiquimod can induce vulvar pain and post-surgical changes can also be painful.

(iv) **Sexual History.** A history of a new sexual contact may suggest a possible sexually transmissible infection such as genital herpes. On the other hand, the complaint of pain may be the presentation of a psychosexual dysfunction, including dyspareunia, relationship problems, fear of pregnancy, or physical abuses.

(v) **Urinary and Fecal Incontinence.** Some women may be embarrassed to complain or are ignorant in seeking treatment for urinary or fecal incontinence. Vulvar irritation and pain may arise from the leaking urine and/or fecal materials.

What are the Common Conditions Causing Pain in the Vulva?

The common vulvar conditions that may present with a complaint of pain includes:

(i) Infectious — Bartholin abscess, Genital herpes, *T. vaginalis* vulvitis
(ii) Inflammatory — lichen planus, lichen sclerosus, endometriosis
(iii) Neoplastic — Paget's disease, squamous cell carcinoma
(iv) Neurological — Herpes neuralgia, spinal nerve compression
(v) Iatrogenic — Topical medications, surgical scars (including episiotomy)
(vi) Vulvodynia

Selected Diseases

1. Bartholin Abscess

Bartholin glands are two mucus secretory glands in the posterior parts of the labia minora. It is 0.5 cm in diameter and is usually not palpable. The gland secretion drains through a 2.5 cm duct to the vaginal orifice just inferior to the hymen and maintains the moisture in the vestibule.

The duct of Batholin gland can be blocked by inflammation or trauma, leading to retention of the gland secretion and formation of a Bartholin cyst of varying sizes, usually between 1 and 3 cm in diameter. The cyst is usually asymptomatic and has been estimated to occur in 2% of women between the ages of 20 and 40. If the cyst becomes infected, there is a rapid progression of inflammation with abscess formation and development of an exquisite vulvar pain. Bartholin abscess can develop without the presence of a Bartholin cyst.

Clinical examination reveals Bartholin abscess as a fluctuant, exquisitely tender mass in the posterior portion of the affected side of the vulva. There may be cellulitis of the overlying skin. If it is discharging spontaneously, the abscess is purulent.

E. coli is the most common (40% of cases) single pathogen in Bartholin abscess. The remaining cases are due to polymicrobial infection from opportunistic bacteria such as *Staphylococcus* and *Streptococcus* species. Unlike studies in the 1970s and 1980s, recent studies rarely find sexually transmitted infection such as N. gonorrhea and chlamydia in Bartholin abscess.

Bartholin cyst may be treated with a marsupialization procedure electively, or drainage with a Word catheter. Bartholin abscess requires a surgical incision, irrigation, draining and packing, together with antibiotic treatment.

2. Genital Herpes

Genital herpes in women involves herpetic lesions in the cervix, vagina, vulva, perineum and perianal region. It is predominantly caused by herpes simplex virus (HSV) type-2 (70% of cases) and, less often, by HSV-type-1. The virus is transmitted sexually. Once inoculated, the virus rapidly gains access to the ganglions or the sensory nerve roots.

Clinical entity of a herpetic lesion is due to reactivation of the virus in the skin supplied by the affected nerves. Typically, the cutaneous lesion first appears as a red papule, which then evolves into a clear vesicle with a red base. Subsequently, the vesicle turns into a pustule which then breaks into a shallow ulcer. Adjacent lesions may coalesce and are extremely painful. This is followed by crusting and healing of the ulcers without any scarring. The entire process takes approximately two weeks.

Genital herpes may by subclinical when the lesions are atypical, or asymptomatic. Both subclinical and asymptomatic cases are shedding HSV as in cases with typical herpetic lesions and are responsible for a vast majority of cases transmitting the virus.

Recurrent genital herpes is common because of the frequent reactivation of the virus. HSV type-2 infection is responsible for almost 95% of all recurrent genital herpes, while women infected with HSV type-1 rarely experience recurrence.

Diagnosis of genital herpes can be confirmed by HSV culture of the vesicular fluid, by serology tests or by PCR-based DNA test.

An acute episode of genital herpes is treated with an antiviral agent. Currently available preparations include acyclovir, valacyclovir and famcicyclovir. All these agents share the same active metabolites which inhibit thymidine kinase activity in viral DNA synthesis. The treatment effectively shortens the clinical duration of the lesions. Suppressive therapy may be needed to reduce the frequency of recurrent reactivation of the virus.

Illustration of Some Conditions that Cause Pain down below

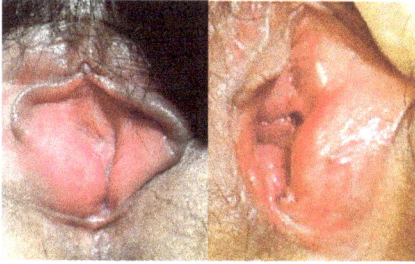

The photograph on the left-hand side shows a case of an uncomplicated Bartholin cyst seen on the mucosal aspect of the right labia minora. The photograph on the right shows a Bartholin cyst that had become inflamed.

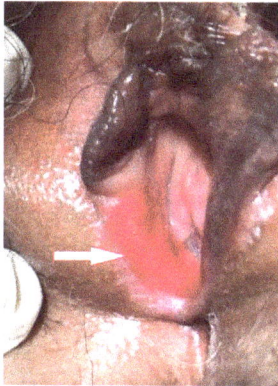

This photograph shows lichen planus presenting as a red lesion (white arrow) on the introitus.

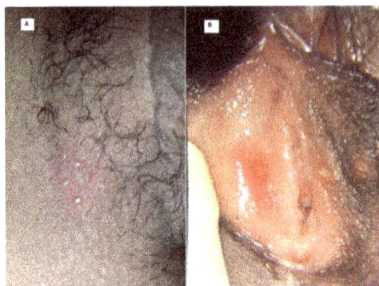

This woman complained of a severe pain in the vulva and acute retention of urine. The photograph shows herpetic vesicles on the cutaneous aspect of the vulva (A) and ulcers on the mucosal aspects of the labia minora and periurethral region (B).

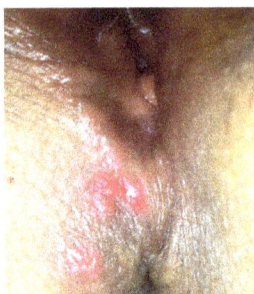

This woman gave a history of recurrent vulvar pain at different locations. This photograph shows red papules on the perineum. Vesicles at the surface of the papules had broken to form shallow ulcers. She had recurrent hepetic lesions.

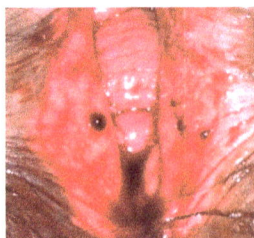

This 40-year-old woman complained of severe pain in the vulva during menstruation. This photograph was taken during the menstrual phase. It shows endometriotic nodules on the mucosa of the labia minora.

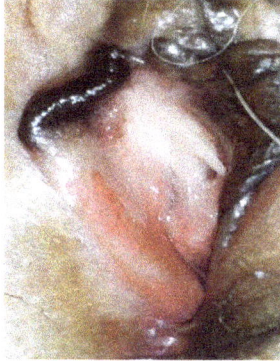

This woman complained of a provoked pain at the vulva. The photograph shows menopausal atrophic vulvo-vaginitis.

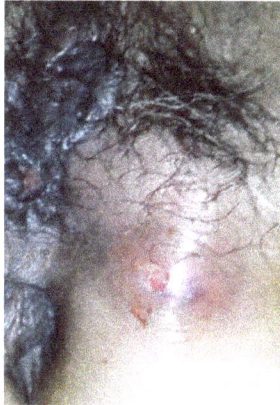

This 48-year-old woman developed an acute pain in the vulvar area over one week. It was painful at rest, on sitting and walking. The photograph shows an inflamed and edematous vulva skin with an abscess. This abscess was not located at the vulva majora as expected in the case of Bartholin abscess. This was a case of pararectal abscess.

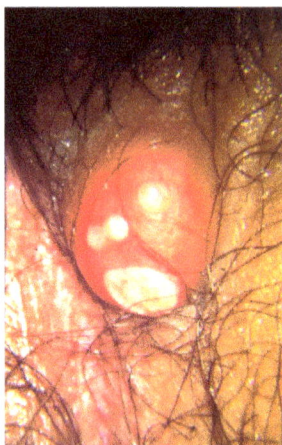

This photograph shows a tumor on the labial majora of a 55-year-old woman. The tumor ulcerations caused severe pain of a recent onset in this patient.

CASE 15 — A LUMP DOWN BELOW

A 50-year-old woman complains of a lump down below.

- What other symptoms are important for reaching a diagnosis?
- What are the common conditions causing this symptom?

What Other Symptoms are Important for Reaching a Diagnosis?

"A lump down below" is a common complaint in gynecology clinic. The lesion may be arising from the vulva, urethra, vagina, cervix, uterus or anus. Several symptoms may reveal or point to the diagnosis of the lesion.

(i) Persistence of the lump: A mass that is persistent in one position is more likely a lesion in the vulvo-perineo-anal region. A mass that appears on exertion or with physical activities and disappears on resting is suggestive of utero-vaginal prolapse. A mass that appears on defecation is suggestive of prolapse of hemorrhoid or rectum.

(ii) Pain: A lump that is painful or is tender is most probably an inflammatory lesion or a superimposed infection in a non-inflammatory lesion, such as a Bartholin abscess, or a vulvar hematoma.

(iii) Bleeding: A lump associated with vaginal bleeding in a woman in the reproductive age group is likely an endometrial or cervical polyp. Vulvo-vaginal condyloma and cancer can also present with bleeding.

(iv) Discharge: A lump with a discharge suggests a cyst, abscess or a tumor.

(v) Urinary and/or fecal incontinence: Utero-vaginal prolapse is often associated with stress incontinence of the urine and/or fecal materials.

What are the Common Conditions Causing this Symptom?

The common conditions presenting as a lump down below can be classified according to anatomical sites:

  (i) Uterus: Uterine or uterovaginal prolapse, endometrial polyp.
 (ii) Cervix: Cervical polyp, cervical cancer, cervical leiomyoma.
(iii) Vagina: vaginal prolapse (cystocoele), urethrocoele, enterocoele, rectocoele, vault prolapse, Gartner duct cyst, vaginal tumor.
 (iv) Vulva: Bartholin cyst, epidermal inclusion cyst, mucous cyst of vestibule, Skene duct cyst, sebaceous cyst, lipoma, fibroma, endometriosis, hematoma, genital warts, vulvar cancer.
  (v) Perineum: Hidradenoma (accessory breast tissue), condyloma
 (vi) Perianal: Hemorrhoids, condyloma, ano-rectal prolapse, ano-rectal cancer.

Selected Diseases

1. Uterine Prolapse

This is also commonly referred to as pelvic organ prolapse ("POP"). With increased life expectancy, up to 70% of elderly women are found to have some degree of uterine prolapse and 30% of women have symptoms of a bulge in the vagina.

Anatomically, the horizontally lying upper vagina and uterus are situated superior to and are actively supported by the levator ani muscles. They are further supported by the ligamental complex from uterosacral-cardinal ligaments, pubocervical fascia and rectovaginal septum. Defect in this support complex can arise from neuro-muscular damage during pregnancy and childbirth.

Ligamento-muscular atrophy following estrogen deficiency of menopause and neuropathy caused by some conditions such as diabetes mellitus, further weaken the uterine support system. Consequently, the uterus descends into the vagina. The prolapse is worsened by long-term increased intra-abdominal pressure in women who have chronic cough and constipation or who is obese.

The symptoms of uterine prolapse vary from no symptoms to a feeling of fullness in the vagina, a dragging sensation in the vagina, low sacral backache, lower abdominal discomfort, sexual difficulty and urinary and/or fecal dysfunctions.

The extent of uterine prolapse is classified into four stages: stage-1 refers to any descent of the cervix up to 1-cm proximal to the hymen; stage-2 refers to further descent of the cervix up to 1-cm distal to the hymen; stage-3 refers to descent beyond 1-cm distal to the hymen; and stage-4 refers to prolapse of the entire uterus with the fundus staying below the hymen, also termed procidentia.

Treatment of Uterine Prolapse

(A) *Non-surgical management*

    (i) Pelvic floor (Kegel) exercise — improved pelvic floor muscle tone may improve stress incontinence of urine but does not improve uterine prolapse.

    (ii) Vaginal pessary — successful support depends on pelvic floor muscle tone and introitus diameter. It is contraindicated in the presence of acute pelvic inflammatory disease or in women with recurrent vaginitis.

(B) *Surgical management*

    (i) With concomitant hysterectomy

        (a) Abdominal approach: (Laparotomy, or laparoscopic, or robotic)

        (b) Sacrocolpopexy: a piece of polypropylene mesh is applied to the upper vagina and cervix and attached to the sacral promontory. It provides a durable repair and maintains the length of vagina. Both the subjective and objective success rate for prolapse correction is more than 80%.

(c) Vaginal approach: this is preferred to abdominal approach for shorter recovery time and low complication rates. There are four common procedures:

- Sacrospinous ligament fixation: permanent sutures are used to attach the vaginal apex to the sacrospinous ligament, 1–2 cm medial to the ischial spine.
- High uterosacral ligament fixation: the strong uterosacral ligaments are shortened and attached to the apex of the vaginal cuff.
- Iliococcygeus fascia suspension: the vaginal cuff is attached to the obturator internus fascia and iliococcygeus fascia.
- Vaginal mesh repair: the attractive idea of combining the low surgical morbidity of vaginal surgery with the durability of polypropylene mess in vaginal mesh repair fell into disrepute due a high postoperative complication rate in mesh erosion, vaginal pain and dyspareunia.

(ii) Without concomitant hysterectomy
  (a) Desire to conserve the uterus

  - Hysteropexy: abdominal approach of sacral hysteropexy is performed in a similar manner as above, without a hysterectomy. Similarly, vaginal sacrospinous hysteropexy can be performed.
  - Manchester repair: this procedure includes a partial trachelectomy, suspension of the uterus using the shortened uterosacral ligaments, and an anterior colporrhaphy.

  (b) Unfit for long surgery

  - Le Fort colpocleisis: this is a vaginal obliterative procedure achieved by excising a patch of anterior and posterior vaginal wall mucosa and suturing together the corresponding cut edges. This is usually performed together with a tight perineorrhaphy for additional support.

2. Cystocoele and Rectocoele

These conditions are the prolapse of the mid-portion of vagina. The vagina is divided into three portions by the anatomical support structures. The upper vagina shares the same support complex as the cervix and uterus and the prolapse of the upper vagina (vault prolapse) is treated in the same way as an uterine prolapse. The distal vaginal is strongly supported by its tight adherence to the urethra and pubis symphysis anteriorly, levator ani-laterally, and perineal musculature posteriorly. The mid-portion of the vagina derives weak support from attachment of paracolpium to the arcus tendineas laterally, pubocervical fascia anteriorly, and rectovaginal fascia posteriorly. Anterior or lateral or both anterior and lateral fascia defects allow the bladder to protrude into the mid-portion of vagina forming a cystocoele. Similarly, a rectovaginal fascia defect allows the rectum to protrude into the vagina, forming a rectocoele. A rectocoele is typically seen as a pocket in the lower vagina just above the level of anal sphincter.

Mild cystocoele and rectocoele have no or little symptoms. In moderate or more severe cystocoele, the patient complains of a bulge in the vagina and there may be urinary dysfunctions such as stress incontinence, difficulty in voiding and sensation of incomplete voiding.

The main symptoms of rectocoele are sensation of a bulge in the vagina, a lump in the introitus and difficulty in defecation. Very often, the patient says that she has to perform a digital splinting of the posterior vaginal wall to pass motion.

The severity of mid-portion vaginal prolapse is graded from 0–4 by physical examination.

Grade 0–Normal position for each respective site;
Grade 1–Descent half way to the hymen;
Grade 2–Descent to the hymen;
Grade 3–Descent half way below the hymen;
Grade 4–Maximal descent possible from each site.

Treatment of Mid-portion Vaginal Prolapse

(A) *Cystocoele*

   (i) Anterior colporrhaphy: repair of central pubocervical fascia defect
   (ii) Paravaginal repair: repair of lateral defect at the arcus tendineas
   (iii) Anterior colporrhaphy and paravaginal repair for combined central and lateral defects
   (iv) Anterior and/or paravaginal repair combined with urethral suspension surgery for stress incontinence of urine

(B) *Rectocoele*

Posterior colporrhaphy is achieved by closing the pararectal fascia over the rectum.

Illustration of Some Conditions that Present as a Lump down below

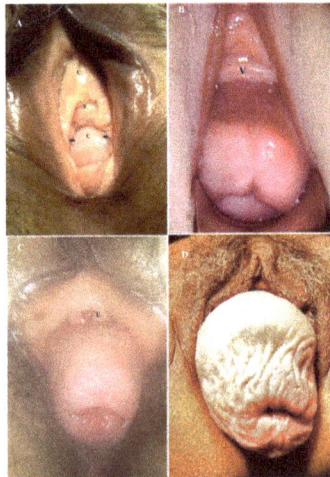

These photographs show different extent of uterine prolapse:

(A) stage-1; (B) stage-2; (C) stage-3; and (D) stage-4 (procidentia).

In panel (A), the arrows identify the hymen. U = urethral meatus; V = vagina; C = cervix.

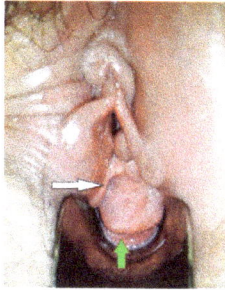

This woman was asymptomatic when she was found to have a grade-1 cystocoele (pointed out by the green arrow). The white arrow identifies the hymen.

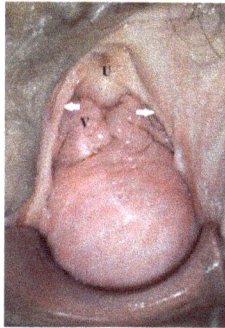

This woman complained of a lump down below for 2 weeks. The lower portion of the vagina (marked "v") was well supported by the adherence to urethra and the pubic symphysis. The arrows mark the hymen. This illustrates a case of cysto-coele.

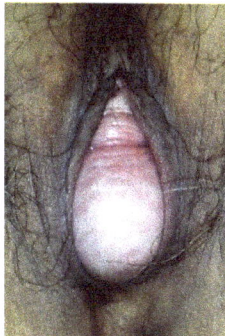

This 60-year-old woman complained of a lump down below after walking for a short distance for 3 weeks. This photograph shows a bulge of mid-portion of vagina extended beyond the hymen, a grade-3 cystocoele.

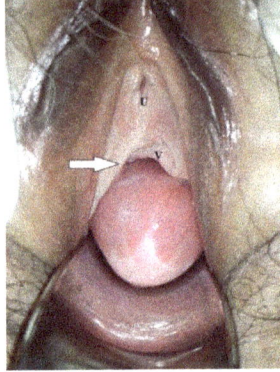

This photograph shows a woman who presented with a lump down below. She had undertaken a hysterectomy some years previously. The anterior vagina (marked "V") was well supported. This illustrates a case of vaginal vault prolapse.

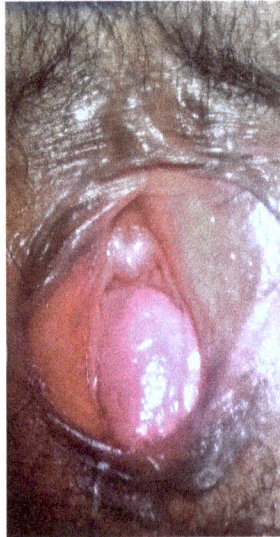

This 50-year-old complained of a painless lump down below. She had chronic constipation and the lump was always more severe when she tried hard on passing motion. This photograph shows a grade-2 rectocoele.

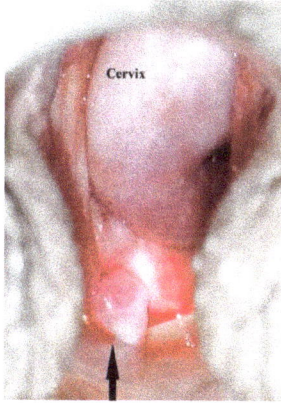

This photograph shows a Gartner Duct Cyst (arrow) situated postero-lateral to the cervix. This is a benign cyst from the embryological remnant mesonephric duct.

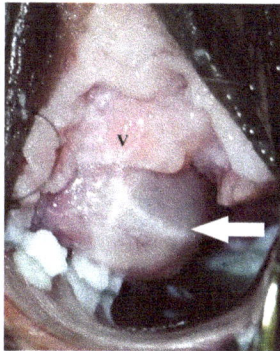

This photograph shows a vaginal cyst (white arrow) seen as a lump down below in a 43-year-old woman. "V" identifies the anterior vaginal wall.

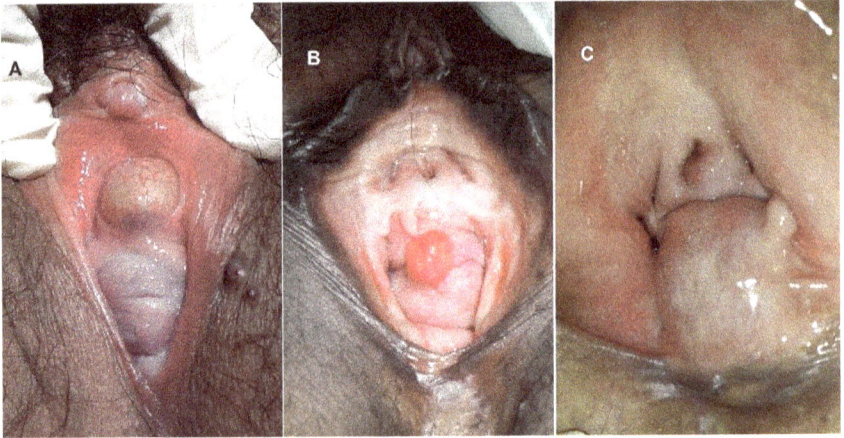

These photographs show vaginal lumps:

Panel (A): Skene gland cyst; (B) a vaginal polyp; and (C) a vaginal mucocoele.

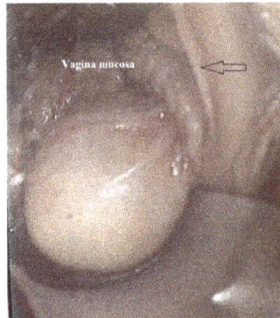

This photograph shows a vaginal cyst. The hymen remnant is marked by open arrow. The cyst is seen to have arisen from the vagina mucosa as seen by the rugae structures.

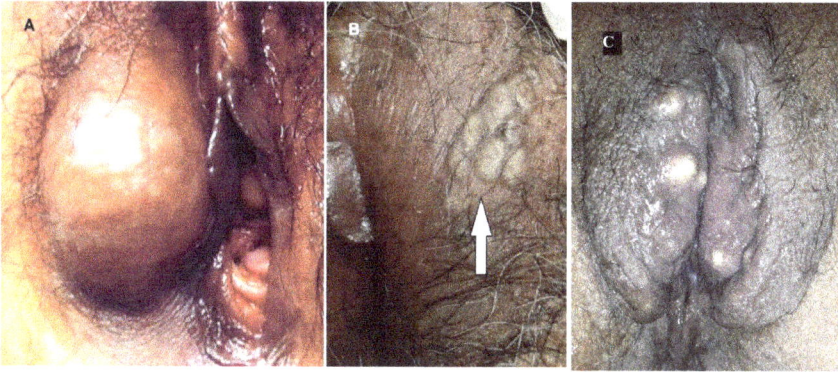

These photographs show vulvar lumps: (A) A large lipoma on the right sided labia majora; (B) and (C): Fordyce spots on the labia majora (white arrow): these are sebaceous cysts of no significance other than cosmetic concerns or fear of being sexually transmitted diseases.

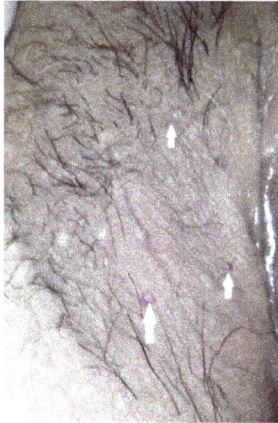

These small red-purplish papules on the vulva majora are angiokeratoma of Fordyce (white arrows). They are vascular papules with hyperkerotosis on the surface skin. They are benign skin lesions.

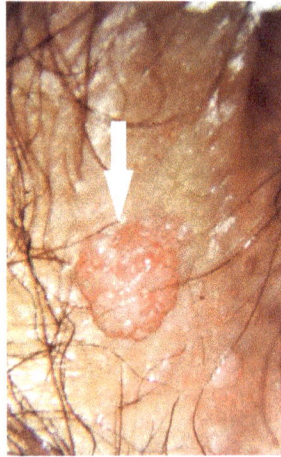

This woman's complaint of a lump down below was explained by a cutaneous wart (white arrow).

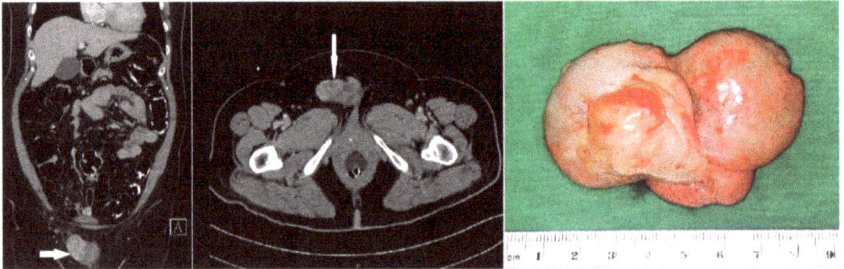

This 65-year-old woman was found on a CT scan on the pelvis to have an 8-cm mass in the vulva (white arrows). She had no symptoms. A soft but firm mass was palpable deep in the subcutaneous compartment of the vulva. This photograph shows a well circumscribed bilobed soft fibroid-like tumor. Histopathology confirmed it a fibromyoblastoma, a benign neoplasm of soft tissue or viscera.

CASE 16 — URINARY INCONTINENCE

A 45-year-old woman complains of leaking of urine on coughing.

- How is the symptom of urinary incontinence evaluated during history taking?
- How can the symptom be evaluated on physical examination?

How is the Symptom of Urinary Incontinence Evaluated during History Taking?

Urinary incontinence is defined as involuntary loss of urine causing a hygienic and/or socio-psychological problem to a woman. The prevalence is estimated to be 1 in 13 for women between 20- and 39-years old; 1 in 7 among 40–59-years old; 1 in 4 among 60–79-years old; and 1 in 3 among women above 80-years old. Symptom evaluation with a detailed history is essential for developing a rational approach to the management of urinary incontinence.

(i) **An experience versus a disorder** — The most fundamental part of symptom evaluation is to determine if urine leaking is an occasional phenomenon that a woman acknowledges during a physician's routine enquiry or survey, or if it is a symptom that a woman seeks consultation from a physician. It is estimated that more than 50% of women never voice their problem of urinary incontinence to a physician. By the time that a woman volunteers the symptom, it is likely that the leak is a significant clinical disorder.

(ii) **Inconvenience versus distress** — Many women manage their urinary incontinence efficiently by trying to pass urine more frequently, by fluid restriction, or by wearing a sanitary pad. The symptom is a mere inconvenience with little impact on their quality of life. On the other end of the spectrum, a woman may suffer a loss of physical activity, compromises sexual life, has great difficulty in maintaining the standard of personal hygiene, or experiences great emotional distress with the experience of urinary incontinence. A number of questionnaires are available for assessing the severity of urinary incontinence, such as Urinary Distress Inventory-6 and Incontinence Impact Questionnaire (IIQ)-7.

(iii) **Provoked versus unprovoked leaks** — Urinary incontinence on provocation, such as by coughing, has a distinct pathophysiology as compared with unprovoked incontinence from enuresis, overflow incontinence and vesicovaginal fistulae. There are a number of well recognized conditions that provoke urinary incontinence, such as coughing, sneezing, laughing, physical activities, brisk walking, housework, sexual intercourse, and others.

(iv) **Other bladder symptoms** — Dysuria is a hallmark of cystitis and/or urethritis which, by increasing the detrusor irritability, may cause incontinence of urine. Urgency and urge incontinence is indicative of an intrinsic detrusor instability. Day frequency and nocturia are non-specific but are often encountered in women with bladder disorders and a number of other systemic illnesses, including diabetes mellitus.

(v) **Rectal symptoms** — Women with urinary incontinence from pelvic floor disorder often has concomitant fecal incontinence.

(vi) **Uterovaginal symptoms** — Uterine and vaginal prolapses often present together with urinary incontinence.

How can the Symptom be Evaluated on Physical Examination?

Physical examination includes three components:

(i) *General Pelvic Condition*
- A speculum examination may reveal a pool of urine in the vagina.
- Pelvic masses — mass compression on the bladder may result in or aggravate the symptom of urinary incontinence
- Urogenital atrophy from estrogen deficiency
- Uterine prolapse, cystocoele, rectocoele
- Urethral diverticulum.

(ii) *Focused Neurological Examination*
- General mental state and gait
- Strength, sensation and deep tendon reflexes of the lower extremities
- Pudendal nerve integrity: sensation of the perineum and perianal area to light touch and needle pricking, the anal wink pelvic floor reflex on stroking the anal canal with a cotton swab.

(iii) *Urinary Incontinence Tests*
- Bladder neck/urethral hypermobility test: with the patient in dorsal lithotomy position and the examining table in parallel to the floor, a lubricated sterile cotton swab is inserted through the urethra. Hypermobility is present if, on patient's Valsalva maneuver, the angle of the swab stick increases from 0° to more than 30°.
- Stress test: lying in dorsal lithotomy position and with an almost full bladder, the patient is asked to cough. Direct visualization of leaking of urine from the urethral meatus is diagnostic of urinary incontinence.

- Marshall-Bonney test: in cases of a positive stress test, a Marshall-Bonney test can be performed by inserting the index and second finger into the vagina and press onto the two sides of bladder neck to support of the proximal urethra. The patient is then asked to cough. Absence of leaking of urine with this test is confirmative of stress incontinence from hypermobility of the urethra.

It is important to note that failure to demonstrate leaking of urine during physical examination does not refute the diagnosis of urinary incontinence. In some cases, leaking of urine is dependent on the patient's posture and the stress test may have to be repeated with the patient in a different position, including on standing up. Other tests such as a pad test using a urine coloring agent (bladder methylene blue, oral phenazopyridine, etc.) may be useful for confirmation of urinary incontinence.

Selected Diseases

1. Genuine Stress Urinary Incontinence (GSI)

GSI is involuntary leaking of urine during provocation which raises the intra-abdominal pressure. Typically, the amount of urine leaking is small. Bladder symptoms such as frequency, urgency and dysuria are usually absent. It affects 15% to 60% of women, depending on the age of the population, but less than half of these women seek medical attention.

In GSI, leaking of urine occurs because the intra-vesicle pressure exceeds the urethra-vesicle pressure gradient during stress situations. In normal physiological state, urinary continence during stress situations is maintained by three mechanisms:

(i) *Voluntary closure of pelvic floor muscle*: contraction of levator ani muscle elevates proximal urethra and bladder neck, tightens the supportive connective tissue fascia, and elevates the perineal body.

(ii) *The adherence of the mid portion of the urethra to the pubic bone* by the pubocervical fascia stabilizes the urethra.

(iii) *The striated muscles of distal urethral sphincter* close the distal urethra.

The resultant effect of these three mechanisms maintains the proximal urethra and bladder neck in the retro-pubic position and a higher intra-urethral than the intra-vesicle pressure at rest. On provocation, both the retro-pubic proximal urethra and the bladder are exposed to the same effect of elevation in intra-abdominal pressure. The higher intra-urethra-vesicle pressure gradient remains unchanged and continence of urine is achieved.

The muscular structure of the pelvic floor and pubo-cervical fascia are exposed to mechanical and neurological traumas from pregnancy and childbirth, particularly in multiparous women, and to degenerative changes after estrogen withdrawal during menopause. These changes result in hypermobility of the urethra and bladder neck. During a stress situation, the proximal urethra and bladder neck rotate out of retro-pubic position and the loss in the intra-urethra-vesicle pressure gradient leads to leaking of urine.

GSI may be complicated by concomitant urge incontinence in what is often termed a mixed urinary incontinence. Symptomatology and physical examination are poor discriminators of GSI, urge incontinence and mixed incontinence. Specific investigations with urodynamic studies allow the bladder function to be objectively evaluated for understanding the pathophysiology of the compliant.

The key components of urodynamic studies relevant to incontinence include:

(i) *Uroflometry* measures the volume of urine voided per unit of time, i.e. the flow rate. Urine flow rate is the function of detrusor contractility, urethral resistance and abdominal muscle straining. It measures bladder outlet obstruction without specific diagnostic information on the etiology of the obstruction. In normal cases, it follows a narrow Bell shape curve with a maximum flow rate of 15–20 mL/s and a voiding time of 15–20 seconds. Of clinical significance, a low flow rate is predictive of a prolonged period of catheterization post-surgery for incontinence.

(ii) *Cystometry* measures bladder capacity, compliance, and the presence of phasic contractions during the filling phase of bladder function. The intrinsic detrusor activity can be detected in the subtracted pressure channel where the intra-abdominal pressure is subtracted from the intra-vesical pressure. The normal bladder capacity is 500–600 mL. The first bladder sensation occurs between 50–200 mL and the urge sensation typically occurs at 200–400 mL. During the filling phase in a normal physiological state, the intrinsic pressure remains stable. A rise of more than 15 cm water from the baseline is considered abnormal and is seen in urge incontinence.

(iii) *Abdominal (or Valsalva) leak point pressure*: with the bladder filled with 150–200 mL of water, the patient is asked to exert Valsalva maneuver several times with increasing strength. The lowest intrinsic pressure that is recorded for observed intrameatus leaking of urine is the abdominal leak point pressure. A leak point pressure of less than 60 cm water is considered diagnostic for intrinsic sphincter deficiency.

The treatment of GSI includes: pelvic floor physiotherapy, anti-incontinence devices, medications and surgery.

(i) *Pelvic floor physiotherapy.* Contraction of the pelvic floor muscles, both the levator ani and pubococcygeus, can be achieved voluntarily by drawing in or lifting up movements as if the voiding or defecation is temporarily stopped without using the abdominal, buttock or inner thigh muscles. These exercises improve the tone and strength of the muscles. When the intra-abdominal pressure is raised, contraction of these muscles stabilizes the hypermobile urethra and helps the urethral shutting pressure. It may take 12 weeks of exercises before its benefit is recognizable while the maximum benefit is reached after six months of the program. In women with mild GSI without intrinsic sphincteric deficiency, a cure rate of 80% has been reported.

Pelvic floor exercises can be augmented with the use of weighted vaginal cones to provide a sensory feedback on the desired strength of muscle contractions or with biofeedback using electronic and computer devices to provide audio- or visual information on muscle contractions.

(ii) *Anti-incontinent devices.* Pad and garment for urine absorption protect the skin and give comfort for patient to continue with their normal activity. They can be used as a temporary measure before definitive surgery or as an adjunct for cases where surgery fails to completely resolve the incontinence.

Urethral occlusive devices are available to compress the urethra for stopping urine leakage. The available single use preparations include the Impress Softpatch (UroMed Corporation, Needham, Mass.), the Reliance Urinary Control Insert (UroMed Corporation, Needham, Mass.), the FemAssist (Insight Medical Corporation, Boston, Mass.) and CapSure Shield (Bard Urological, Covington, Ga.), and the Introl Bladder Neck Support Prosthesis (UroMed Corporation, Needham, Mass.)

(iii) *Medications.* Alpha agonists (midodrine, pseudoephedrine) may increase the sphincteric urethral tone and improve urinary incontinence subjectively in 20% to 60% of women.

Tricyclic anti-depressants, such as imipramine and amitriptyline, possess central and peripheral anti-cholinergic effects, as well as alpha adrenergic effects. Clinically, it relaxes bladder muscles and increases the urethral sphincteric tone. It has been shown to be useful in women with mild GSI and mixed stress and urge incontinence.

Duloxetin is a serotonin/norepinephrine reuptake inhibitor known to increase the output of pudendal motor nucleus of the sacral segment with an increase in urethral muscle tone and closure pressure. It has been shown to be useful in improving the symptoms and frequency of incontinence in women with mild-moderate GSI.

(iv) *Surgery*. The objective of surgery is to increase the urethral outlet pressure. Numerous surgical techniques are available but the main approaches in wide use today include:

(a) Bladder neck suspension: Burch retro-pubic urethropexy restores the intra-abdominal position of the vesico-urethral junction and proximal urethra by attaching the paravaginal fascia to the pectineal lines. It can be done through an open surgery or laparoscopically. The success rate of 90% at 5-year follow up has been reported. This procedure is possible only in women with sufficiently mobile vagina. On the other hand, it does not correct cystocoele, rectocoele and introitus deficiency.

(b) Midurethral sling operation: in the Tension-free Vaginal Tape (TVT) procedure, a synthetic tape is inserted, through a small suburethral vaginal incision, into the space of Retzius and brought out of the abdominal wall suprapubically. Instead of suspending the mid-urethra through the anterior abdominal wall, a similar procedure with the tape placed on the mid-portion of the obturator canals inside the thigh creases at the level of the clitoris is known as the transobturator sling (TOT or TVT-O). TVT has a cure rate of 85% at 10-year follow up. TVT-O appears to have a comparable outcome as TVT.

(c) Periurethral bulking therapy: synthetic materials, bovine collagen and some autologous substances can be injected into the periurethral tissue to inflate the submucosal tissue of the bladder neck and sphincter. This relatively non-invasive technique increases the urethral pressure. Its efficacy in treating GSI is inferior to sling operations and repeated therapy is required.

(d) Artificial urinary sphincter (AUS) placement: AUS, such as AMS 800, mimics biological bladder sphincter. This is rarely performed for treatment of urinary incontinence in women.

2. Urge Urinary Incontinence

Urge incontinence of urine is an uncontrollable passing of urine associated with a sudden onset of an intense urge to void.

Provocative factors may be absent or may be situational such as on seeing the toilet, reaching the door on returning home, turning on of washing machine, etc. Associated symptoms of frequency and nocturia are common.

The pathophysiology of urge incontinence is complex and involves detrusor myopathy, neuropathy, or combination of both. In the normal state, the bladder relaxes and the intra-vesicle pressure remains low during the filling phase. When the bladder is sufficiently distended, the intrinsic detrusor activity increases to generate the first sensation of urge for voiding. In women complaining of urge incontinence, the abnormality in detrusor activity results in a premature initiation of micturition reflex with a sudden and strong urge and uncontrollable voiding.

Treatment

Urge incontinence from detrusor instability is not curable but the symptoms can be controlled by several approaches.

(a) *Life Style Changes.* Behavioral modification is recommended as the initial attempt to improve the symptoms of urge incontinence.

   (i)   Dietary changes: control the consumption of caffeine, alcohol, nicotine, or spicy or acidic foods.
   (ii) Weight control: reducing obesity by weight loss of 5% to 10% has been reported to improve the symptoms of incontinence.
   (iii) Bladder schedule re-training: planned voiding at increasing lengthening intervals, often supplemented with relaxation techniques; distraction strategies and/or deep breathing exercises may assist in symptom control.
   (iv) Pelvic floor exercises have been recommended as part of the conservative management of urinary incontinence. It has a moderate efficacy in young and middle aged women with stress incontinence. Its role in urge incontinence is not well demonstrated.

(b) *Drug Therapy.* The treatment of urge incontinence in women is largely drug therapy with an aim to improve the bladder compliance and capacity. Changing the life style may improve the symptoms of urge incontinence at the initiation of drug therapy but it does not increase the rate for stopping drug therapy.

(i) Anticholinergic agents: these drugs are significant for their clinical benefits in increasing the bladder capacity and threshold for initiating involuntary contractions. They are the mainstay of medical treatment of urge incontinence in women.

Oxybutynin has been reported to reduce the episodes of urge incontinency by 80% and a total continent rate of 50%. Tolterodine is an antimuscarinic agent which reduces muscle contractions in the urinary tract selectively and has a similar clinical efficacy as oxybutynin on continence rate but with less severe side effects of dry mouth, dry eyes and constipation. Solifenacin (Vesicare) is a competitive muscarinic receptor antagonist with a clinical inhibitory effect on bladder smooth muscle contraction.

(ii) Botolinum toxin: clinical experience shows that intradetrusor injection of onabotulinum toxin A via cystoscopy repeatedly over a 12-week period results in a high continent rate with fewer systemic side effects compared to anti-cholinergic agents, except a higher rate for urinary retention and urinary tract infection.

(iii) Estrogen therapy is often recommended for treatment of urinary incontinence in postmenopausal women. Systemic estrogen replacement has a low success rate for urinary incontinence.

Illustration of Urodynamic Changes in Women with Urinary Incontinence

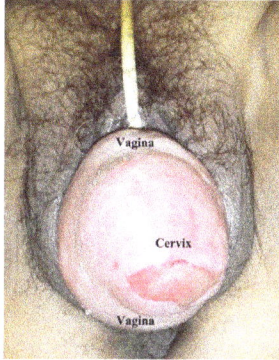

This woman was coping well with urinary frequency and incontinence for two years. One day, she developed acute retention of urine. The photograph shows the severe uterine prolapse which was a probable explanation of her failure of micturition.

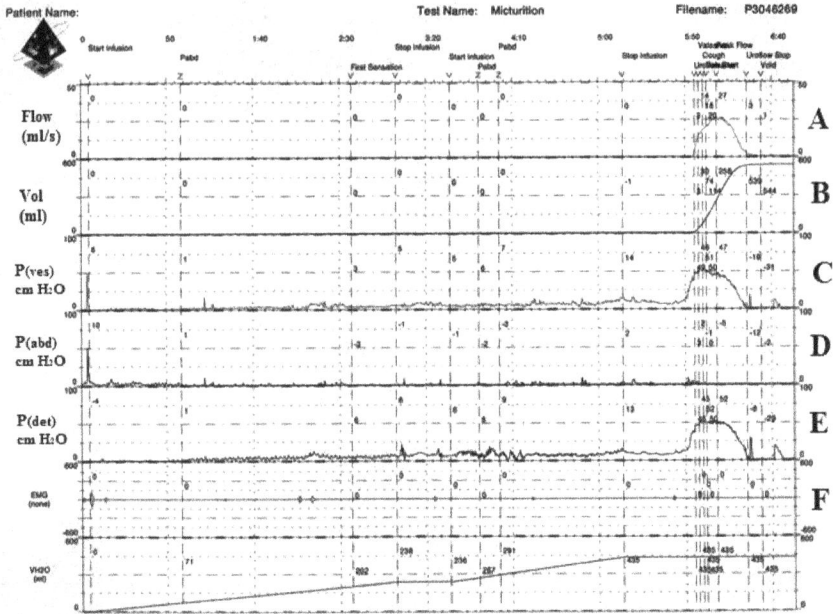

This chart shows the findings on urodynamic study of a normally functioning bladder.

Row-A shows the flow rate in mL/second.
Row-B shows the volume of urine voided (mL).
Row-C: the intra-vesicle pressure (cmH_2O).
Row-D: Intra-abdominal pressure (cmH_2O).
Row-E: Detrusor pressure (cmH_2O) is calculated by subtracting intra-abdominal pressure from the intra-vesicle pressure.

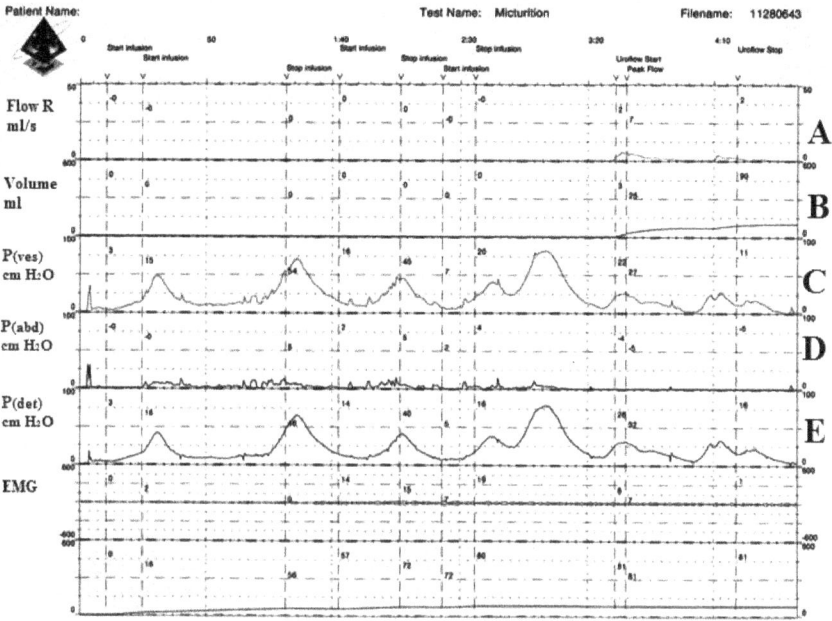

This chart shows the findings on urodynamic study of a case of detrusor instability. The detrusor pressure (Row-E) is shown to be fluctuating (unstable) throughout the bladder filling phase.

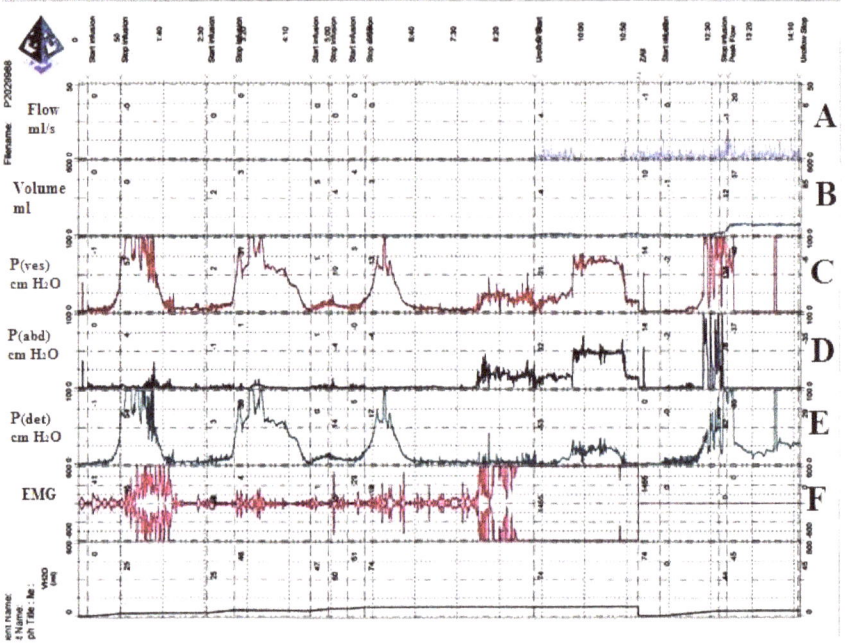

This chart shows a case of detrusor hyperreflexia in which the unstable detrusor pressure was caused by uninhibited detrusor muscle contractions (Row-F). In some cases, this condition is caused by neurological disorders. The patient complains of urinary frequency, urgency and incontinence.

CASE 17 — ACUTE ABDOMINAL PAIN

A 26-year-old nulliparous woman complains of a lower abdominal pain of sudden onset.

- What history would suggest that she has a gynecological condition?
- What are the common gynecological causes?
- What assessment of this patient would you perform initially?

What History would Suggest that she has a Gynecological Condition?

Acute abdominal pain located below the level of umbilicus is also referred to as acute pelvic pain. This is a pain of sudden onset in a previously well person. It is the presenting complaint in 1.5% of all office consultations and 5% of emergency room consultations. Acute abdominal pain can arise from reproductive, urinary or intestinal systems, or musculoskeletal structures. A detailed history of the pain is essential for its correct diagnosis:

(i) **Location of Pain.** Acute appendicitis may have a sharp pain at the right iliac fossa of the abdomen but is often associated with a history that the pain had been periumbilical initially. In contrast, gynecological cause of pain tends to start and stay at the lower abdomen.

(ii) **The Characteristic of the Pain.** Pain from acute appendicitis tends to be constant and is progressive in severity, and aggravated by physical movements. Pain from ureteric calculus is associated with the well-known clinical expression of "moan, groan, stone." On the other hand, pain from many gynecological causes is described as "cramping," similar in character to menstrual pain.

(iii) **Specific symptoms suggestive of a gynecological cause of pain include:**

  (1) Temporal relationship to menstruation: mid-cycle, pre-menstrual, menstrual, or immediately postmenstrual;

  (2) Menstrual abnormality: heavy menstruation, irregular menstruation or amenorrhea

  (3) New onset vaginal discharge

  (4) New onset dyspareunia

  (5) New sexual partner

  (6) Recent application of intrauterine contraceptive device or gynecological surgery.

It is noteworthy that a history of urinary frequency and/or dysuria, diarrhea, constipation or dyschezia, and abdominal bloating, while suggestive of urinary tract or bowel conditions, do not exclude a gynecological cause of pain.

What are the Common Gynecological Causes of Acute Pelvic Pain?

Common gynecological causes of acute abdominal pain can be categorized by the associated history:

(1) **Pain at mid-menstrual cycle.** Mittelschmerz.

(2) **Pain before menstruation.** Ovarian cyst complications, endometriosis.

(3) **Pain with heavy menstruation.** Fibroids, adenomyosis, endometriosis, endometritis, miscarriage.

(4) **Pain with irregular menstruation.** Miscarriage, ectopic pregnancy, endometritis, endometriosis.

(5) **Pain with amenorrhea.** Inevitable miscarriage, ectopic pregnancy, ovarian cyst.

(6) **Pain with a vaginal discharge.** Pelvic inflammatory disease, tubo-ovarian abscess.

(7) **Pain after IUD/gynecological surgery.** Pelvic inflammatory disease, tubo-ovarian abscess, endometritis, ectopic pregnancy.

What Assessment of this Patient would you Perform Initially?

The initial assessment of a patient complaining of an acute abdominal pain should include:

(i) **Cardiovascular stability.** The first step of clinical assessment is to perform a rapid survey for fever, shock, hemorrhage, dehydration and cardiac decompensation. Where necessary, resuscitative measures should be immediately implemented to stabilize the patient's condition.

(ii) **Obtain a detailed history** of the pain, menstrual history and relevant medical history.

(iii) **General physical examination.** A complete physical examination must be carried out.

(iv) **Abdominal examination.** Observe for any swelling and movement of abdominal wall with respiration, identify the location of point of maximum pain and evidence of peritonism (guarding and rebound tenderness), palpate for abdominal masses, and auscultation for bowel sounds.

(v) **Pelvic examination.** A vaginal examination is performed to inspect for vaginal discharge and to obtain samples for bacteriological investigations. The presence of cervical excitation pain is noted and the status of the cervical os ascertained. This is followed by a bimanual examination of the pelvis to assess the site and degree of tenderness and presence of any masses.

(vi) **Rectal examination.** To assess any fecal impaction, tumor or blood in the ano-rectum and to complete the pelvic examination transrectally.

(vii) **Urinary β-HCG** for pregnancy detection.

(viii) **Bedside ultrasound scan** of the pelvis to detect pregnancy, uterine abnormalities, adnexal masses, or fluid in the pelvis.

(ix) **A full blood count** for anemia and leukocytosis.

(x) **A urine analysis** for pyuria and hematuria.

Selected Diseases

* Ectopic pregnancy
* Miscarriage
* Ovarian cyst

1. Ectopic Pregnancy

Ectopic pregnancies are gestations located outside the uterine cavity, most commonly in the fallopian tube (97%) and, of these, 80% are in the ampulla region. Ectopic pregnancy can also occur at the uterine cornua, cervix, ovary and abdominal viscera.

Ectopic pregnancy reportedly occurs in 1% of all conceptions and accounts for 5% of pregnancy-related maternal mortality in developed countries. It is the leading cause of maternal mortality occurring during the first trimester of pregnancy. More than 90% of deaths from ectopic pregnancy are caused by hemorrhage.

The great majority of these women do not have any apparent risk factors for ectopic pregnancy. Epidemiological data shows that the risk for ectopic pregnancy is higher among women with the following conditions:

(i) *Tubal Structural Abnormalities*

* *Prior salpingitis and pelvic inflammatory disease.* Incidence of tubal damages increases with frequency of PID, being 13% after 1 episode, 35% after 2 episodes and 75% after 3 episodes. It is noteworthy that chlamydia infection of the genital tract is often

asymptomatic and may explain why many women diagnosed with ectopic pregnancy do not seem to carry a recognizable risk factor.

- *Previous ectopic pregnancy.* Recurrence rate of ectopic pregnancy is 10% to 25%.
- *Tubal surgery (including tubal occlusive procedures) and re-anastomosis.* Almost 50% of pregnancy after tubal occlusive procedure for permanent contraception is ectopic. Other tubal surgeries also carry an increased risk of tubal pregnancy.

(ii) Tubal Motility Anomaly

- *Progestogen-only contraceptive pills*
- *Intrauterine contraceptive device.* Generally, IUD prevents pregnancy and thus reduces the prevalence of ectopic pregnancy among the users. However, if an IUD user becomes pregnant, the risk of ectopic gestation is estimated to be 10%.
- *Cigarette smoking.* Human and animal studies show that cigarette smoking reduces the motility of the fallopian tube. The relative risk of ectopic pregnancy is 1.6 to 3.5 for smokers as compared with non-smokers.

(iii) High Maternal Age

Compared to women between 15–24-years old, women between 35–44-years old have a 3-fold increased risk of ectopic pregnancy.

(iv) IVF Pregnancy

IVF pregnancies have an ectopic pregnancy rate of 4.5%.

Symptoms

1. The triad of ectopic pregnancy, pain, amenorrhea and abnormal vaginal bleeding occurs in 50% of all cases. Individually, acute

abdominal pain is present in 98% of cases, amenorrhea in 75% of cases, and abnormal vaginal bleeding in 60% of cases.
2. Pregnancy symptoms: nausea and vomiting, dizziness, fatigue, constipation.
3. Shoulder tip pain
4. Recent onset of dyspareunia

Clinical Signs

1. Unstable hemodynamic state with hypovolemic shock and a tender rigid abdomen can occur, though less frequently now because of earlier diagnosis with modern medical care. This is a surgical emergency as the symptoms are indicative of a ruptured ectopic gestation with intra-abdominal hemorrhage.
2. Localized peritonism: lower abdominal tenderness and rebound tenderness, and cervical excitation pain.
3. Adnexal tenderness, more intense on one side.
4. A palpable adnexal mass. Absence of an adnexal mass on pelvic examination does not exclude an ectopic pregnancy.

Differential Diagnosis

1. Complications of early pregnancy:
   - Spontaneous abortion
   - Incomplete abortion
   - Threatened miscarriage
   - Molar pregnancy
2. Complications of ovarian cyst:
   - Ruptured corpus luteal cyst
   - Ovarian torsion
3. Menstrual disorders:
   - Dysmenorrhea
4. Acute appendicitis
5. Urinary tract infection

6. Other causes of hemorrhagic shock
7. Other causes of hypovolemic shock

Diagnosis of Ectopic Pregnancy

1. *High index of suspicion* for ectopic pregnancy is needed when one is dealing with a woman presenting with an acute abdominal pain during the reproductive era.

2. *Urinary and serum β-HCG test for pregnancy.* Sensitive urinary assays can detect β-HCG at a low level (25 mIU/mL) to indicate an early pregnancy.

   Serial quantitative serum β-HCG assays may show a subnormal rise in its level. In early pregnancy, serum β-HCG doubles in concentration every 48–72 hours. However, this phenomenon is unreliable for the diagnosis of ectopic gestation. More importantly, serum quantitative β-HCG is used for its discriminatory zone for ultrasound imaging study.

3. *Transvaginal ultrasound scan.* A discriminatory zone of β-HCG for an intrauterine gestational sac is 700–1000 mIU/mL and for an intrauterine pregnancy is 1500–1800 mIU/mL. This discriminatory zone is raised to 2500 mIU/mL if multiple gestations are expected such as in women undergoing *in vitro* fertilization program. An empty uterus on a transvaginal ultrasound scan when serum β-HCG level is above the discriminatory zone is an indication of an ectopic pregnancy.

   Transvaginal ultrasound imaging sometimes detects an ectopic pregnancy as a tender adnexal mass or, less frequently, a gestation sac containing a fetal pole with cardiac pulsations outside the uterus. A ruptured ectopic pregnancy is suspected if the fallopian tube is seen to be filled with blood or free fluid. An unruptured tubal pregnancy is sometimes seen as a ring-like echogenic structure outside the uterus. An interstitial ectopic pregnancy is seen as a gestation located eccentrically in the upper part of the uterus and is surrounded by a thin (<5 mm) myometrial mantle.

4. *Laparoscopy.* Laparoscopy is the gold standard procedure for diagnosis of ectopic pregnancy. It carries a sensitivity of more than 95%. It provides the exact location, size and integrity of the ectopic gestation. More importantly, it is diagnostic of other pelvic conditions that mimic ectopic pregnancy such as PID and ovarian cyst.

Treatment

1. Expectant treatment

Application of sensitive diagnostic test has led to the observation that almost 25% of cases of early ectopic pregnancies regress spontaneously. Expectant treatment is an acceptable option with close follow up to demonstrate objective evidence of resolution by β-HCG assays and ultrasound imaging. Successful outcomes have been reported in more than 70% of these selected patients.

The criteria for selecting patients to be treated expectantly are:

- Asymptomatic
- Initial β-HCG titers below 1000 mIU/mL
- Small gestation (≤4 cm in greatest dimension)
- No evidence of rupture
- Hemodynamically stable
- Fully compliant with follow up
- Willing to accept the potential risks of tubal rupture

2. Medical treatment

Medical treatment of ectopic pregnancy has gained an increasing popularity in the last three decades as it avoids the morbidity of surgery. It is suitable for ectopic gestation in the fallopian tube but is particularly attractive for cases where the ectopic gestation is on the cervix, uterine cornua or ovary, as surgery in these cases often involves loss of the organ.

Methotrexate, an anti-folate known to be highly cytotoxic to trophoblastic tissue, has established as an effective treatment of ectopic pregnancy for patients who fulfill the following criteria:

- Hemodynamically stable
- Gestation size ≤4 cm at its greatest dimension on ultrasound imaging
- Absence of fetal cardiac activity on ultrasound imaging
- No evidence of tubal rupture
- β-HCG level less than 5000 mIU/mL
- Fully compliant with treatment and follow-up care

The following groups of patients are not suitable for methotrexate therapy of ectopic pregnancy: known hypersensitivity to methotrexate, on breastfeeding, liver disorders, hematological dysfunctions, renal dysfunctions, and immunosuppression.

Methotrexate is administered as 50 mg/m^2 in a single intramuscular injection and the serum β-HCG level is monitored on days 4 and 7 after the injection and weekly thereafter until it becomes negative. The success rate of treatment exceeds 90%.

The side effects of methotrexate are largely gastrointestinal, such as nausea and vomiting, gastric pain and diarrhea. Other symptoms include stomatitis and dizziness. Almost every patient experiences at least one episode of abdominal pain, most often 2 to 3 days after the injection. When the pain is prolonged, an ultrasound scan may be performed to exclude rupturing of the ectopic pregnancy.

3. Surgical treatment

Laparoscopy is the recommended approach to surgical treatment of ectopic pregnancy, leaving laparotomy to cases where the hemodynamic condition of the patient is unstable, or for uterine resection for interstitial and corneal pregnancies. Effective surgical techniques include linear salpingotomy, segmental salpingectomy, and salpingectomy for tubal gestations, uterine resection for cornua pregnancy, and salpingo-oophorectomy for ovarian pregnancy. The subsequent fertility rate is similar regardless of the types of surgical treatment, but is influenced by the state of the contralateral fallopian tube and concomitant pelvic adhesions or endometriosis.

- Salpingotomy: In this fertility sparing surgery, a 1–2 cm linear incision is made over the gestation location on the antimesenteric border of the fallopian tube. The gestation sac is removed with aqua-pressure and the bleeding arrested with electrocoagulation.

    Persistent trophoblastic tissue following salpingotomy has been reported in 5–15% of cases. Most of these cases resolve spontaneously. However, complication with bleeding or rupture of the tube may occasionally occur. Patients treated with salpingotomy should be followed up with weekly serum β-HCG assay which usually becomes negative within 2–3 weeks. Plateauing or rising β-HCG levels is an indication for additional methotrexate therapy or surgery.

- Segmental salpingectomy: Isthmic tubal pregnancy is often associated with severe damages beyond salvage. Ectopic gestations located in the mid-portion of the fallopian tube are amenable to segmental salpingectomy where the involved segment of the tube is excised. Immediate or interval tubal re-anastomosis can be performed for fertility preservation.

- Salpingectomy: Total salpingectomy by dissecting the tube along the mesosalpinx from the fimbrial end to the uterine junction is the preferred surgery for a damaged tube in a ruptured ectopic pregnancy, in recurrent ectopic pregnancy on the same tube, and in patients who are hemodynamically unstable. This is also the treatment of choice for patients who want to avoid the morbidities of persistent trophoblastic tissue that are seen in some cases treated conservatively.

4. Anti-D prophylaxis

Rhesus blood group should be determined and Rhesus negative women should be given anti-D immunoglobulin injection to prevent isoimmunization.

Illustration of Ectopic Pregnancies

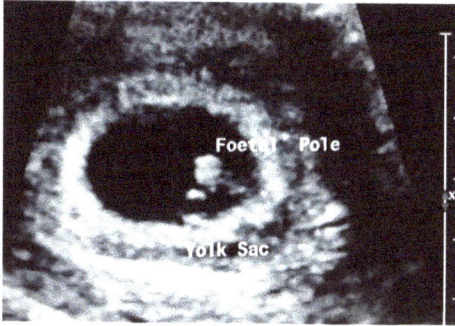

This photograph of an ultrasound scan of the uterus shows a gestational sac with fetal pole and the yolk sac from an early viable pregnancy. This finding excludes ectopic pregnancy as the incidence of co-existing intrauterine and extrauterine gestations is lower than 1 in 40,000 pregnancies.

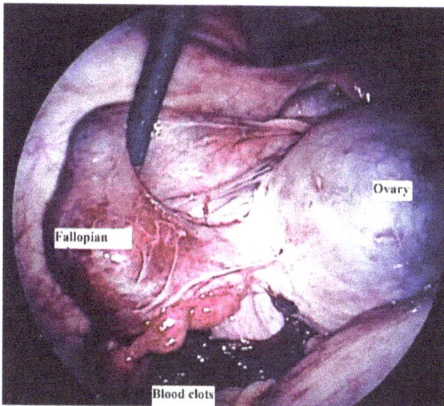

This woman with sudden onset of acute abdominal pain was found on a laparoscopy to have a left-sided fallopian tubal pregnancy. The fallopian tube was intact. The ovary had a corpus luteum.

A 43-year old woman who had an ectopic pregnancy of seven weeks gestation. Serum β-HCG was 3173 IU/L. A transvaginal ultrasound scan showed that the uterus was normal in size and the endometrium measured 15 mm in thickness, without a gestational sac. There was a 19 mm corpus luteum in the right ovary. In the medial aspect of the ovary was an irregular cystic area of $9 \times 5 \times 5$ mm with a cystic area $1 \times 1 \times 1$ mm, resembling a yolk sac. No obvious fetal pole or heart pulsations seen.

The patient was treated with methotrexate 50 mg/m^2 intramuscularly on 11 March 2015. The trend of serum β-HCG was monitored. A rise in β-HCG to 6332 three days after treatment was noted before it started to decline and reached a negative value of 3.1 IU/L on 11 April 2015, as shown in the chart below.

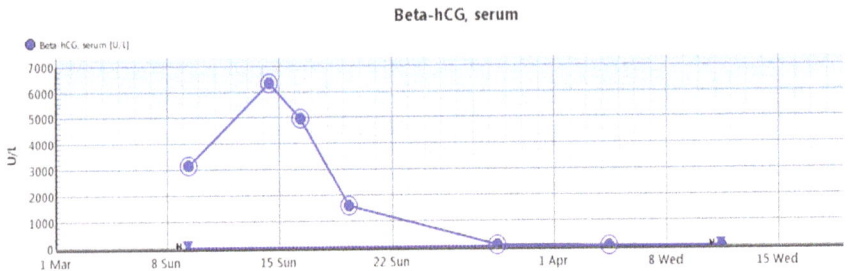

Ectopic pregnancy treated with intramuscular injection of methotrexate.

2. Miscarriage

Miscarriage, also known as spontaneous abortion, refers to pregnancy loss before 20 weeks gestation and is confined to clinically diagnosed pregnancies by biochemical tests and ultrasound imaging. It occurs in 5–15% of all pregnancies and the incidence increases with the increasing maternal age. Miscarriage accounts for 4% of pregnancy-related maternal mortality in developed countries.

Causes

(i) *Embryopathy*

This accounts for 80–90% of all first trimester miscarriages as more than 90% of chromosomally and cytomorphologically abnormal embryos are terminated spontaneously. The most common chromosomal aberration is trisomy, with trisomy 16 accounting for a third of all cases.

(ii) *Maternal systemic medical disorders*

- Diabetes mellitus
- Severe hypertension
- Renal disease
- Systemic lupus erythematosus
- Thyroid dysfunctions
- Infection: (e.g. rubella, cytomegalovirus CMV, and mycoplasmal, ureaplasmal, listerial, toxoplasmal infections)

(iii) *Maternal luteal deficiency*

(iv) *Maternal uterine anomaly*

- Congenital: Septated uterus, didelphys uteri,
- Acquired: Intrauterine adhesions, fibroids, cervical incompetence

(v) *Drugs/toxins*

- Alcohol
- Tobacco
- Cocaine

Clinical Presentation

Miscarriage occurs in two clinical forms.

1. Pre-symptomatic miscarriage

This is also termed a missed abortion. The patient is asymptomatic but the pregnancy is found to be non-viable on ultrasound imaging, either as an empty intrauterine gestation sac or an embryo with no cardiac pulsations.

2. Clinical miscarriage

The patient presents with vaginal bleeding and abdominal pain during pregnancy. There are four stages of spontaneous miscarriage:

(i) *Threatened miscarriage.* This is defined as vaginal bleeding without passage of pregnancy tissue and the cervical os remains closed. Almost 25% of pregnancies are complicated by at least one episode of threatened miscarriage and half of these cases result in spontaneous miscarriage. The amount of bleeding is generally not heavy and the abdominal pain is mild and cramping. Clinically, the patient's general condition is stable. Abdomen is soft and not tender on examination. On pelvic examination, blood in the vagina and cervical os is evident. The cervical os is closed and excitation pain is absent. The uterus is gravid size, soft and not tender.

(ii) *Inevitable miscarriage.* This is diagnosed when vaginal bleeding is associated with a dilated cervical os as it denotes that the progressive process of spontaneous miscarriage is unavoidable. The bleeding is heavier and the pain is more severe than that seen in threatened miscarriage.

(iii) *Incomplete miscarriage.* Vaginal bleeding associated with passing or passed products of conception is an incomplete miscarriage. The cervical os may be open or closed. The bleeding is heavy or life-threatening. The pain is severe in the lower abdomen and may radiate to the back or the lower genital tract.

(iv) *Complete miscarriage.* The products of conception have completely been passed and the vaginal bleeding and abdominal pain subsided. The cervical os is closed and the uterine cavity is empty on ultrasound imaging.

Differential Diagnosis

The differential diagnosis in any woman of reproductive age presenting with a history of acute abdominal pain and vaginal bleeding should include:

(i) *Pregnancy-related disorders*

- Ectopic pregnancy
- Miscarriage
- Molar pregnancy

(ii) *Menstrual disorders*

- Abnormal uterine bleeding
- Dysmenorrhea
- Endometriosis

(iii) *Ovarian cyst*

- Ovarian cyst
- Ovarian torsion

(iv) *Acute appendicitis*

(v) *Urinary tract infection*

Diagnostic tests

(i) Urinary pregnancy test
(ii) Serum β-HCG assay
(iii) Ultrasound imaging

Urinary pregnancy is highly sensitive in the diagnosis of pregnancy. Serum β-HCG allows differential interpretation of ultrasound imaging in the detection of an ectopic pregnancy.

High resolution transvaginal ultrasound scan provides accurate information on the location and size of pregnancy as well as the fetal cardiac activity. Ultrasound findings of the different stages of the miscarriage include:

(i) Missed abortion: irregular gestation sac with absence of an embryo (anembryonic) or an embryo with no demonstrable cardiac activity. Subchorionic hematoma may or may not be present.

(ii) Threatened miscarriage: the gestation sac is appropriate for period of pregnancy. If embryo is present, it is of appropriate dimensions for the gestation and cardiac activity is demonstrable. There may or may not be subchorionic hematoma.

(iii) Inevitable miscarriage: the gestational sac may or may not be regular or collapsed and cardiac activity may or may not be detectable.

(iv) Incomplete miscarriage: gestation sac is irregular or collapsed. Blood may be seen in the uterine cavity with solid materials.

(v) Complete miscarriage: the uterus is empty. The diagnosis of a complete miscarriage has to be weighed against an ectopic pregnancy.

Management

(i) *Threatened miscarriage*

1. Inform the patient on the viability of the fetus
2. Expectant management for 14 days
3. If bleeding stops, continue routine antenatal care
4. Re-assess the condition if the bleeding gets worse.

(ii) *Miscarriage*

1. Expectant treatment:
   - Confirm diagnosis of miscarriage
   - Informed consent on treatment options
   - Watch for 14 days if the patient has low risk for severe bleeding, except
     — Late first trimester
     — Coagulopathy/on anticoagulation

     — Cannot take transfusion of blood

     — Bad obstetric history: recurrent miscarriage, antepartum hemorrhage, stillbirths

- Analgesia
- Information on when to attend emergency treatment
- If bleeding stops within 7–14 days, perform a pregnancy test three weeks after
- Re-assess with an ultrasound scan if:
  - Bleeding does start within 14 days
  - Worsening bleeding/pain not stop by 14 days

2. Medical treatment

- Confirm the diagnosis of missed abortion or incomplete miscarriage
- Informed consent on options of treatment and adverse effects of medicines
- Vaginal misoprostol 800 mg single dose
- Analgesia and antiemetics
- If bleeding does not start within 24 hours, return for individualized care
- If bleeding/pain settles within 14 days, perform a urinary pregnancy test
- Return for individualized care if vaginal bleeding persists after 14 days or pregnancy test after three weeks is positive

3. Surgical treatment

- Confirm diagnosis
- Informed consent
- Manual vacuum aspiration of the uterus under local anesthetics or in theatre under general anesthesia.

4. Anti-D prophylaxis: Rhesus blood group should be determined and Rhesus negative women should be given anti-D immunoglobulin injection to prevent isoimmunization.

3. Ovarian Cysts

Ovarian cysts are fluid or semi-fluid filled structures in the ovaries. They are found on ultrasound scan of the pelvis in almost all premenopausal women and in up to 18% of postmenopausal women. They induce a lot of anxiety among women and their physicians because of the cystic presentation of ovarian malignancy and the potential risk of complications in some benign ovarian cysts.

Ovarian cyst can be fundamentally classified into non-neoplastic and neoplastic categories:

1. *Non-neoplastic cysts*

- Cysts of mesothelial origin
- Cysts of follicular origin
- Cysts of inflammatory conditions (endometrioma, tubo-ovarian abscess)

2. *Neoplastic cysts*

- Epithelial — benign cystadenoma
  — malignant cystadenocarcinoma
- Germ cell — mature teratoma (Dermoid cyst)
  — immature teratoma

1. *Non-neoplastic or functional ovarian cysts*

(i) *Follicular cysts*

- Results from failure of ovulation or atresia of partially developed follicles as a consequence of suboptimal LH surge, excessive FSH stimulation or hormonal therapy
- Extremely common and may be multiple
- 3 cm in dimension, rarely exceeds 5 cm
- Unilocular, thin wall with a smooth lining, clear and watery contents
- Can be associated with oligo- or amenorrhea
- Often regress spontaneously

(ii) *Corpus luteal cysts*

- Results from failure of regression of corpus luteum. Most commonly developed after corpus luteam hematoma
- 3–5 cm in dimension
- Complex cyst on ultrasound scan — "ring of fire" appearance from rich blood flow on the periphery of the corpus luteum on Doppler scan
- Lined by luteinized granulosa cells with theca cells in deeper layers
- Dull, unilateral pelvic pain
- Persistent progesterone secretion results in delayed menstruation which may present as continuous vaginal bleeding
- Complications with rupture/hemorrhage later

(iii) *Theca-lutein cysts*

- Results from intense luteinization and hypertrophy of the theca interna cells as a consequence of excessive stimulation from human chorionic gonadotropin (hCG)
- Commonly bilateral
- Usually small but may be multiple and large (up to 20 cm) in hyperestrogenic state such as twins pregnancy, on gonadotrophin treatments (ovarian hyperstimulation syndrome), molar pregnancy and choriocarcinoma.
- Can lead to massive ovarian enlargement termed hyper-reactio luteinalis
- Predisposed to torsion, hemorrhage, and rupture.

(iv) *Luteoma of pregnancy*

- Results from proliferation of luteinized stromal cells
- Androgen secretary in up to 30% of cases, of which 50% develops virilization of the female fetus
- Complex, heterogenous, hypoechoic mass on ultrasonography
- resolves after completion of pregnancy

2. *Neoplastic cysts: Benign variety*

(i) *Benign epithelial neoplasms*

- Differentiated along Müllerian pathway:

  - Tubal: serous cystadenoma, can be sub-classified by morphological appearance:
  - Serous (1–30 cm in diameter, smooth/glistening inner & outer surfaces, clear and water content, histologically single layer of flattened or cuboid cells)
  - Papillary serous (papillae formed of loose fibrous tissue lined by tubal-like epithelium are seen on inner or outer, or both surfaces. Psammoma bodies may be seen in the papillae tissue)
  - Serous adenofibroma (lobulated, hard, knobbly solid mass on the inner cyst wall. Microscopically, they are fibrous tumors containing small cysts or gland-like spaces lined by tubal-like epithelium)
  - Endometrial: endometrioid cystadenoma (very rare, resembling endometrial polyp)
  - Endocervical: mucinous cystadenoma (common, accounting for 20% of benign ovarian tumors. Cystic and lobulated with smooth/glistening surfaces. 15–30 cm, but can occupy the entire abdominal cavity. The cyst ccontent is clear, tenacious mucoid material. Histologically, the cyst is lined by a single layer of columnar cells resembling endocervical epithelium)

- Differentiated along Wolffian pathway:

  - Brenner tumor (uncommon, <2 cm in dimension, smooth and hard. May become cystic in the center, lined by flattened endothelial-like cells, cuboid cells or mucus secreting cells. Almost always benign)
  - Mesonephroid tumor (exceptionally uncommon, usually solid fibromatous)

(ii) *Germ cell neoplasm*

Mature cystic teratoma (Dermoid cyst)

- Forms 10–20% of all ovarian tumors and 97% of all ovarian teratomata. It can occur in women of any age but 90% of these cases are found during reproductive years.
- Round or ovoid cyst, 5–15 cm in size and 10% of the cases are bilateral.
- Cyst content is yellowish-brown, greasy. There may be hair, teeth, cartilage or bones (may be specific bones). Cyst lumen contains a hillock-like protuberance known as Rokitansky's tubercle, the nipple or the mammillary body.
- Cyst wall is lined by squamous epithelium. Other tissue types are commonly present: respiratory, GIT, cartilage and bone, thyroid and salivary, neural, etc.

Risk Factors for Ovarian Cysts

- Reproductive age group
- Early menarche
- First trimester of pregnancy
- Personal history of infertility or PCOS
- Intrinsic or extrinsic gonadotrophins
- Tamoxifen
- Personal or family history of endometriosis
- Cigarette smoking
- OCP usage is protective

Clinical Presentation

- Asymptomatic
- Menstrual irregularity
- Dyspareunia
- Pelvic pain (common): the prevalence of ovarian cysts ranged from 3% to 9.5% among women who complain of a new-onset abdominal pain.

- Abdominal bloating and early satiety (common)
- Urinary frequency and dysuria
- Palpable adnexal mass (common)
- Less than 1 in 3 ovarian cysts are detectable on bi-manual examination

Differential Diagnosis of Ovarian Cyst Include the Following

- Polycystic ovarian syndrome
- Paraovarian cyst
- Hydrosalpinx
- Peritoneal cyst
- Tubo-ovarian abscess
- Pedunculated leiomyoma
- Pelvic lymphocele
- Abdominal abscess
- Psoas abscess

Diagnosis

1. Ultrasound scan: This is excellent in detecting enlargement of ovary or part of ovarian tissue. It also provides information on the consistency of the cyst in terms of being cystic, solid or complex cystic-solid nature. The imaging study can be complemented with Doppler blood flow study. These features allow clinical distinction of different types of ovarian cysts. The reported sensitivities and specificities are 88% and 90%, respectively for ovarian malignancy, 92% and 97% for endometrioma, and 90% and 98% for dermoid cysts.

   Ultrasound scan may detect some complications of an ovarian cyst. For example, it may show a twisted vascular pedicle, the "whirlpool sign" during active ovarian torsion, and hemorrhage in a cyst may show the blood as a diffuse reticular "fishnet pattern" or "spider web" appearance. Blood clot can be distinguished from solid cyst component by the absence of demonstrable blood flow on color Doppler ultrasonography.

2. CT Scan: This technology allows detection of enlargement of ovary or ovarian tissue and raises suspicion of malignancy in the presence of ascites, wall/septal thickness >3 cm, or peritoneal, mesenteric, or omental masses. This is particularly called for if cancer is suspected based on ultrasound findings. For determining malignancy, it carries a sensitivity of 90% and specificity of 75%.

3. MRI: It demonstrates enlargement of ovary or ovarian tissue and raises suspicion of malignancy if necrosis is present in solid tissue. Its specificity is superior to ultrasound (73% versus 63%).

4. Serum CA125: In the presence of an ovarian cyst, serum CA125 is a useful adjunct in the assessment of the risk of malignancy. It is elevated in 80% of women with epithelial ovarian cancer in general, and 50% of patients with stage-1 cancer. A levil >35 U/mL in postmenopausal women warrants a concern for ovarian cancer. In the premenopausal patients, elevated levels are associated with many benign conditions, such as uterine fibroids, PID, endometriosis, adenomyosis, pregnancy, and menstruation. The overall sensitivity and false-positive rate of serum CA125 for ovarian malignancy ranges from 50% to 83% and 14% to 36%, respectively.

Complications of ovarian cysts

- **Ovarian torsion:** The incidence is low but may be higher during pregnancy with an estimated rate of 1% to 7%. Ovarian torsion can occur at any age of women but more than 70% of surgically treated torsions occur in women below 30-years old. It is more common (60%) for the torsion to occur in the right ovary. The classical symptoms are sudden onset of severe unilateral lower abdominal pain with a history of worsening over several hours. There may be a low-grade fever. Nausea and vomiting occur in 70% of the patients. The diagnosis is accurate in only 57.8% of cases at the first clinical examination.

Ovarian necrosis is the complication of torsion. Treatment with laparoscopy is successful in one third of patients.

- **Cyst rupture:** The incidence is low and it often follows sexual intercourse, exercise, or pelvic examination. Rupture is more common in corpus luteal cyst which often occurs between days 20 and 26 of a normal menstrual cycle.

  Dermoid cysts may also rupture. The released cyst contents often trigger an inflammatory cascade resulting in peritonitis.

- **Cyst hemorrhage:** A catastrophic intraperitoneal bleed may result from rupture of a corpus luteal cyst, specifically among patients on anticoagulants or with bleeding disorders.

- **Cyst infection:** This results from either ascending genital tract infection as in pelvic inflammatory disease or hematogenous inoculation of bacteria in the ovarian cyst.

- **Dyspareunia:** Ovarian cyst sometimes causes a new onset dyspareunia. The incidence is low. Cervical excitation pain on clinical examination and pain on intercourse is more commonly associated with pelvic inflammatory disease.

- **Ovarian cancer:** The potential of a benign ovarian cyst becoming malignant has not been proved, but malignant change may occur in a small percentage of endometriomas.

Management

Management of ovarian cyst is determined by the symptoms, cyst dimension, suspected pathology and the patient's health condition.

(i) *Premenopausal simple cyst*

- Expectant management is the choice as 50–75% of simple ovarian cyst <6 cm will resolve spontaneously. Cyst resolution is not hastened by the use of oral contraception pills. It is noteworthy that removal of benign cysts does not reduce the mortality from ovarian cancer.

- Tissue diagnosis (fine needle aspiration) is not recommended as the test carries a low sensitivity (25%) and high false-positive rate (73%).

- Laparoscopic ovarian cystectomy is the surgical approach of choice for persistent ovarian cyst.

(ii) *Premenopausal complex or solid cysts*

- Physiological forms of complex ovarian cysts such as corpus luteal cysts often resolve spontaneously, but as a group, many are persistent. One study demonstrated an 8.3% spontaneous resolution rate over 34 months.

- If the diagnostic impression of the cyst is benign, they should be managed conservatively, with serial ultrasounds every two to three months. For a persistent cyst, laparoscopy ovarian cystectomy for histopathological assessment is warranted.

- Comparing laparoscopy to laparotomy in premenopausal women with benign-appearing masses, laparoscopy yielded a low complication rate, decreased operative morbidity, decreased hospital stay, and decreased postoperative pain. Although spillage of the cyst contents is higher among laparoscopy group as compared with laparotomy group for dermoid cystectomy (18% versus 1%), no increase in morbidity was noted.

- When a malignancy cannot be excluded, the patient should be referred to a gynecologic oncologist for a more extensive laparotomy, including staging and exploration of lymph node status.

(iii) *Postmenopausal simple cyst*

- The risk of malignancy is extremely low (<0.1%) for unilocular ovarian cysts <10 cm in diameter. Of these, more than 70% resolved spontaneously. These cysts should be treated with conservative observation as a first-line treatment, with serial ultrasounds and CA-125 levels every two to three months.

- If the cyst increases in size or a high morphology index of malignancy is indicated, surgical evaluation and cyst removal for histopathological diagnosis are mandatory.

- Laparoscopy should be reserved for cysts with a low suspicion for malignancy.

(iv) *Postmenopausal complex or solid cysts*

- Women with a nodular or fixed pelvic masses, CA-125 value >35 U/mL, evidence of metastasis, or presence of ascites should be offered laparotomy by an experienced gynecologic oncologist.
- There is an increased survival and prognosis for women with ovarian cancer managed by gynecologic oncologists.

(v) *During pregnancy*

- Ovarian cysts are detected by routine ultrasound scans in 1–4% of women during the first or second trimester. The majority of these cysts are corpus luteal cysts, of which, more than 95% resolve spontaneously by 20 weeks gestation. They present no risk to the pregnancy.
- Risk of ovarian malignancy is 1 in 12,000 to 47,000.
- Risk of complications such as torsion or rupture ranges from 1% to 6%.
- Thus, first-line treatment remains conservative, with observation and serial ultrasounds.
- For persistent benign-appearing cysts that produce symptoms of pain or mass effect compression on other organs, laparoscopic exploration and cyst removal should be considered.
- If the cyst demonstrates characteristics of malignancy, surgical removal during pregnancy should be undertaken by laparotomy in the second trimester.

Illustration of Ovarian Cysts

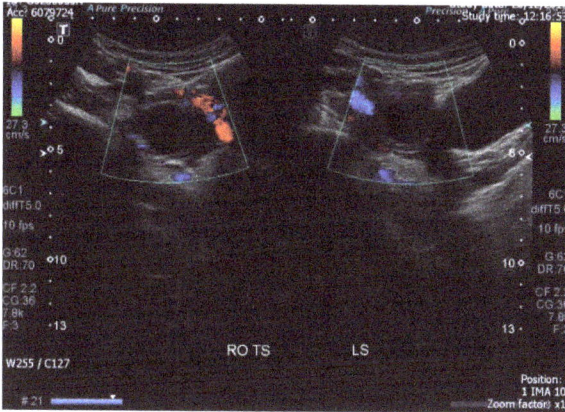

This photograph shows an ultrasound scan with Doppler blood flow study on an ovarian cyst. The intense blood flow at the periphery of the cyst wall in the form of a "ring of fire" is diagnostic of a corpus luteal cyst.

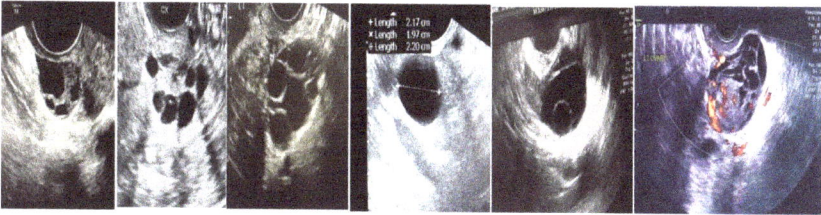

This panel of ultrasound scan photographs shows different types of ovarian cysts.

Panel (1) a dominant follicle; panel (2) polycystic ovarian syndrome with multiple small cystic spaces distributed at the periphery of the ovary; panel (3) a multi-lobulated ovarian cyst; panel (4) an simple-looking inclusion cyst in a postmeno-pausal woman; panel (5) an ovarian cyst with a daughter cyst; and panel (6) a complex appearing cyst with intense "ring of fire" blood flow of a corpus luteal cyst.

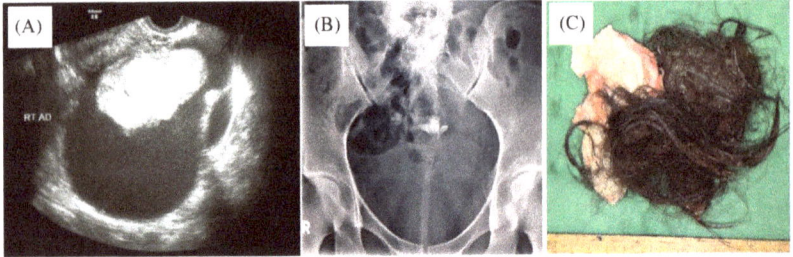

This 25-year-old woman had a large cystic mass in the right ovary. Ultrasound scan (Panel A) shows a cystic mass with a large solid area. Panel (B) shows a plain X-ray illustrating a tooth-like calcification in the mass. Panel (C) shows the opened cystic teratoma with a turf of hair and a piece of irregular bone measuring 4-cm in length. Benign ovarian teratomas or dermoid cysts are the most common germ cell tumors of the ovary. They are the most common benign ovarian tumor in adolescents and young women.

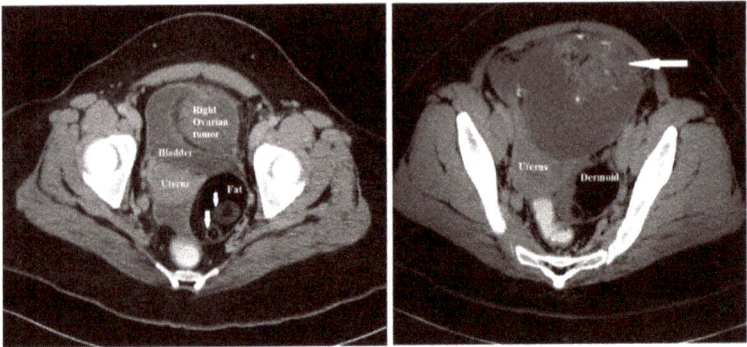

This 30-year-old woman presented to the emergency room with an acute onset abdominal pain. There was an abdominal-pelvic mass to the size of a 20 weeks gestation. This panel of photographs shows two sections of T2 signal MR imaging. The panel on the left shows a left ovarian cyst with fat content and solid components (marked by white arrows), consistent with a dermoid cyst. There was also a right ovarian tumor which on the next section of the MR imaging study shows a large right ovarian tumor with solid material showing calcification, consistent with a teratoma. She underwent a laparotomy and bilateral ovarian teratomas were confirmed. The left ovarian tumor show a grade-1 immature teratoma and the left tumor was a mature teratoma (dermoid cyst). There was spontaneous rupture of the right ovarian teratoma which was the cause of her acute abdominal pain.

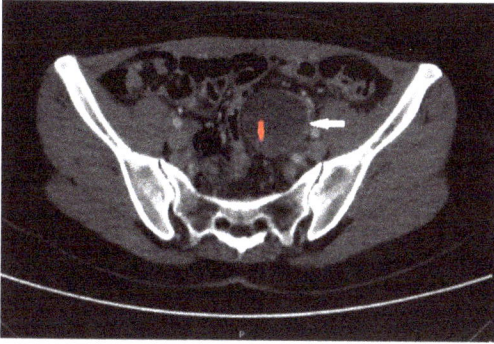

This woman complained of a progressively more severe left iliac fossa pain over 6 hours. This photograph of a section of CT-scan shows a left ovarian cyst of 4.6 cm in diameter (indicated by the white arrow). There were sedimentations in the cyst to suggest a hemorrhage within the cyst (red arrow). She was managed expectantly with analgesia and the cyst resolved spontaneously on the follow up period.

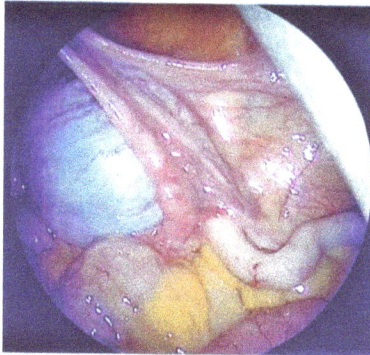

This young woman presented with a sudden onset of right iliac fossa pain and a low grade fever. She underwent a laparoscopy for a suspected acute appendicitis. This photograph shows that the appendix was normal. There was a right ovarian cyst.

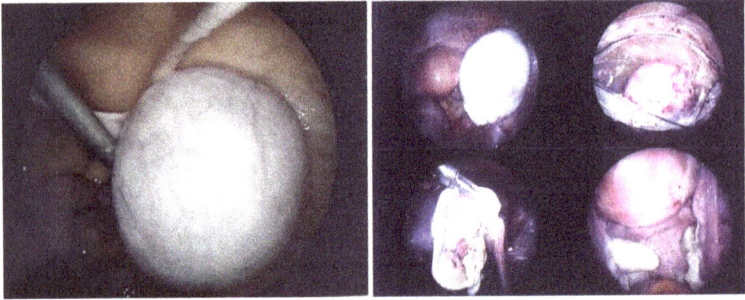

This woman had large ovarian cyst (panel on the left-hand side). A laparoscopy ovarian cystectomy was performed and the intact cyst was captured in a surgical plastic bag for retrieval of the cyst without spillage of cyst contents (panel on the right-hand side).

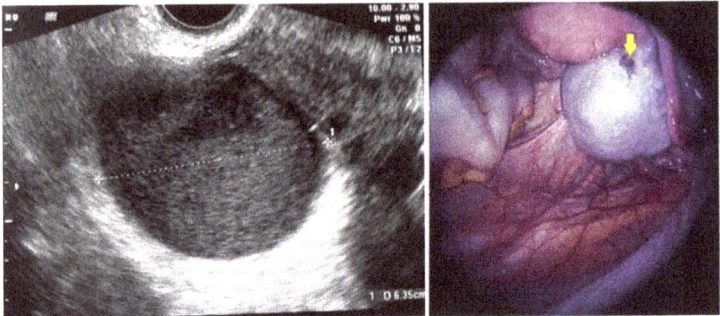

This woman with a short history of abdominal pain was found to have a 6.3 cm right ovarian endometriotic cyst (hyperechoic ultrasound feature). On laparoscopy, endometriotic spot (marked by yellow arrow) was the tell-tale sign of endometriosis in the origin of the ovarian cyst.

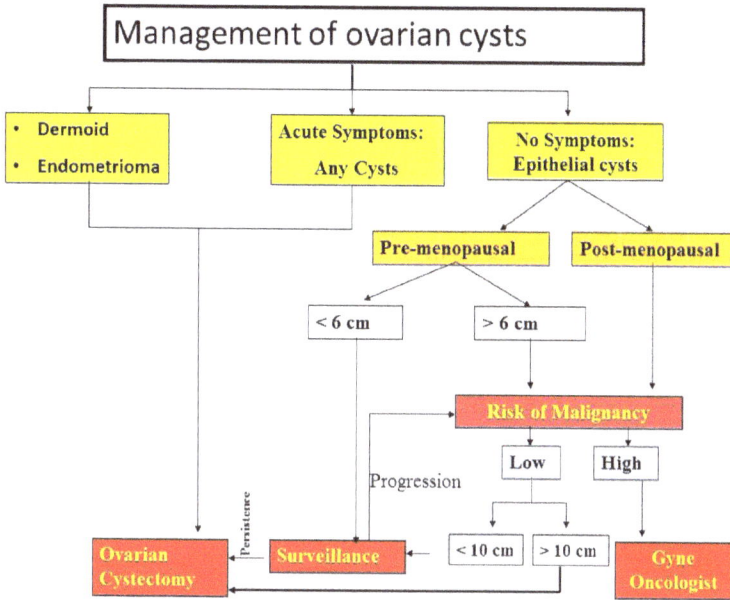

This chart summaries the work-flow of management of ovarian cysts.

CASE 18 — CHRONIC PELVIC PAIN

A 32-year-old woman complains of a lower abdominal pain for the third episode within the last 12 months.

- What are the definition and significance of chronic pelvic pain (CPP)?
- What are the common causes of CPP?
- How should women with CPP be investigated?
- How is CPP managed?

What are the Definition and Significance of Chronic Pelvic Pain (CPP)?

Chronic pelvic pain refers to physically, emotionally and/or psychologically distressing pain, cyclic or non-cyclic, in the lower abdomen for a duration of six or more months, excluding specific dysmenorrhea and dyspareunia. As a general guide, the patient's pain is considered distressing if she volunteers the symptom. In contrast, pain that is elicited on physician's solicitation is unlikely to be a distressing symptom. CPP is a symptom which requires a diagnosis of the underlying disorder.

Population-based surveys from the USA, UK, Australia and New Zealand reported that CPP has a prevalence of approximately 20% among women of reproductive age. The common belief that CPP is commoner in younger than older women has been challenged by the new emerging data which showed that women above 55-years old shared an equally high prevalence of CPP as in younger women. There is no clear evidence of any impact of socio-demographic factors on the prevalence of CPP.

CPP is associated with poor quality of life, low self-esteem, and loss of working hours and capacity, feeling of despair, anxiety, depression, and increased suicide rate. Almost a third of women with CPP never seek medical consultation and 40% are on self-medication. On the other hand, CPP accounts for 40% of gynecological diagnostic laparoscopies.

What are the Common Causes of CPP?

CPP can be a manifestation of diseases of the visceral, neurovascular and musculoskeletal structures in the lower abdomen and pelvis, or psychosocial disorders. These disorders can be categorized as below:

(i) **Gynecological Disorders.** Endometriosis, chronic pelvic inflammatory disease, pelvic congestion syndrome and adhesions.
(ii) **Urological Disorders.** Interstitial cystitis, chronic urinary tract infection, stone and bladder neoplasm.
(iii) **Gastrointestinal Disorders.** Constipation, irritable bowel syndrome, inflammatory bowel diseases.
(iv) **Musculoskeletal Disorders.** Chronic coccygeal pain, pelvic floor myalgia, fibromyalgia.
(v) **Neurological Disorders.** Neuropathic pain, nerve entrapment.
(vi) **Psychosocial Disorders.** Anxiety, depression, post-traumatic stress disorders, physical and sexual abuse.

Community-based study from the UK and New Zealand reported that etiological diagnosis of CPP can be reached in only 50% of cases. Among these, irritable bowel syndrome were diagnosed in 20% of cases, ovarian cysts, endometriosis and pelvic inflammatory diseases were diagnosed in about 7–10%, respectively, and fibroids, adhesions, constipation and back pain were diagnosed in about 5%, respectively.

How should Women with CPP be Investigated?

The main challenge in determining the cause of CPP is the overlapping symptomatology. All patients with CPP should be assessed with an in-depth history and physical examination of the abdomen and pelvis to identify the potential underlying disorders, to direct secondary diagnostic investigations, and for specific specialist referrals for a multidisciplinary management:

- Cyclic intermenstrual pain: Mittelschmerz pain occurs during the mid-cycle following ovulation. The leaking of prostaglandin rich follicular fluid, and sometimes bleeding, causes the localized pain in the iliac fossa or across the lower part of the abdomen.
- Dysmenorrhea/deep dyspareunia/Pelvic nodularity and tenderness: These are the common signs and symptoms of endometriosis.
- Vaginal discharge/dyspareunia/cervical excitation pain/ pelvic tenderness are clusters of signs and symptoms of pelvic inflammatory disease.
- Abdominal pain/dyspareunia/pelvic mass may indicate the diagnosis of ovarian cyst and/or uterine fibroids.
- Dyspareunia/apareunia/dyschezia/Pelvic floor spasm typically reflects pelvic floor myalgia.
- Micturition frequency/urgency/dysuria/Anterior vaginal wall tenderness/normal Pouch of Douglas point to urinary tract infection; interstitial cystitis; painful bladder syndrome.
- Abdominal pain and bloating/pain relieved by defecation/frequent stool/soft stool or diarrhea: are classical signs and symptoms of irritable bowel syndrome.
- Tingling sensation/numbness/history of surgery/tumor treatment: neuropathy; nerve entrapment
- Pain aggravated by movement and or posture/normal pelvis: musculoskeletal disorders.
- Anxiety/depression/normal pelvis: psychosocial disorders.

Laboratory Investigations

• *Microbiological*

Vaginal and/or endocervical swabs for STDs: gonorrhea and chlamydia PCR.

Mid-stream urine for microscopy examination and for bacterial culture of urinary tract infection.

• *Biochemistry*

B-HCG to rule out pregnancy
Serum CA125 in women with new onset of IBS after 50-years of age and in women whose CPP is associated with abdominal bloating, early satiety and frequency of micturition.

• *Hematology*

White blood cell count, ESR

• *STD serology*

Syphilis, Hepatitis B and HIV

• *Imaging studies*

Pelvic ultrasound scan: diagnosis of endometriosis, adenomyosis, fibroids, ovarian cysts and tumors.

Pelvic MRI: indicated for specific diagnosis and is superior to laparoscopy in its sensitivity and specificity for adenomyosis of the uterus and deep infiltrative pelvic tissue.

Surgical Procedures

Laparoscopy

Laparoscopy establishes a diagnosis in approximately 50% of cases of CPP. It carries a very high sensitivity for pelvic inflammatory disease, adhesions, endometriosis and ovarian cysts. It also allows specific therapeutic procedures to be carried out.

Laparoscopy is indicated only after a meticulous evaluation of possible causes of CPP and when the pain control is unsatisfactory on conservative management, including possible psychological intervention.

Hysteroscopy

Hysteroscopy is performed for diagnosis confirmation and therapeutic surgery for endometrial polyps and submucous fibroids after ultrasound imaging studies.

Cystoscopy

This is performed in CPP associated with frequency of micturition, dysuria and microscopic hematuria in whom almost 40% would have interstitial cystitis.

Colonoscopy

Women above 50-years old with a new onset CPP associated with IBS symptoms or a change in bowel habits or blood in stool should undergo a colonoscopic evaluation.

How is CPP Managed?

Management of CPP is complex and, despite a multidisciplinary approach, remains unsatisfactory in a significant proportion of women. The initial management of CPP can be summarized as below:

(i) CPP with an identifiable organic diagnosis: treat the primary diagnosis appropriately.
(ii) CPP with dominant gynecological symptoms: analgesia and ovarian suppression with either GnRH analogue, progestogens, or combined oral contraceptive pills.
(iii) CPP with dominant IBS symptoms: anti-spasmodic medications such as merbeverine, dietary modifications, and psychological intervention.
(iv) CPP with dominant bladder pain symptoms: dietary modifications, bladder training and pelvic floor physiotherapy, amitriptyline and anti-spasmodic medications.
(v) CPP with dyspareunia without organic diagnosis: pelvic floor physiotherapy, psychological therapy.
(vi) CPP with fibromyalgia/neuropathy: pelvic floor physiotherapy, gabapentin, amitriptyline, psychological therapy.

Illustration of Some Conditions Causing Chronic Pelvic Pain

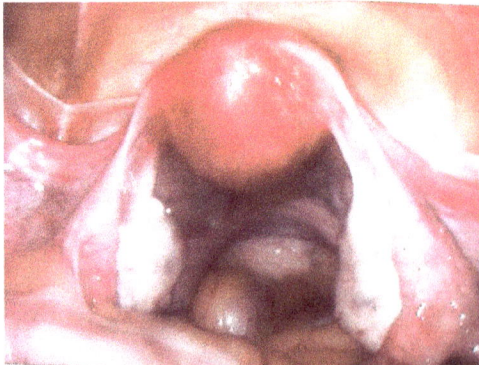

Laparoscopy for chronic pelvic pain often finds no pelvic anatomical abnormalities as shown in this photograph.

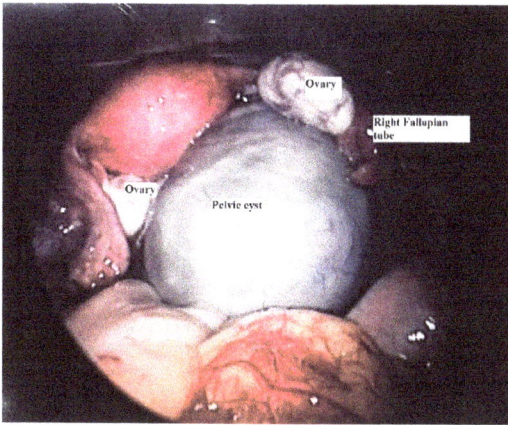

This photograph of a laparoscopy shows the pelvic structures as labeled and a large pelvic cyst. The patient experienced chronic pelvic pain for 6 months before the pain progressed thereafter that prompted her seeking of medical attention. The cyst was confirmed to be a large benign pelvic peritoneal cyst.

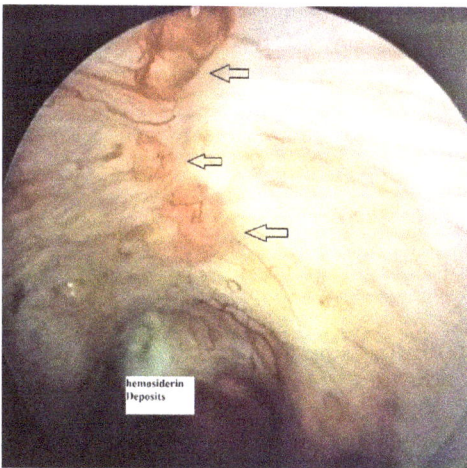

This photograph of a laparoscopy shows deposits of fresh endometriosis (indicated by arrows) and hemosiderin deposits of old endometriosis on the pelvic peritoneum.

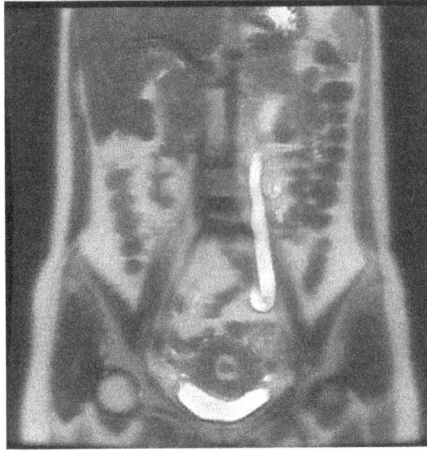

This photograph of a MRI section demonstrates gross hydroureter on the left-hand side. The distal ureter was obstructed by deep infiltrative endometriosis. She experienced chronic pelvic pain and was treated repeatedly for recurrent cystitis, with aggravation of pain during menstruation.

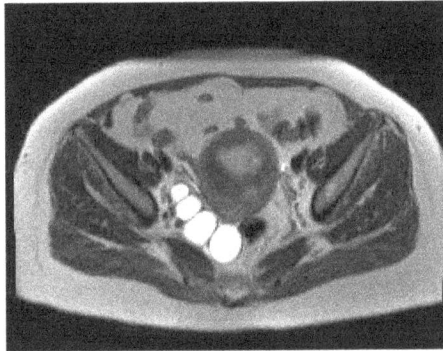

This photograph of a section of MR imaging study of the pelvis in a woman with chronic pelvic pain shows hydrosalpinx of the right fallopian tube from chronic pelvic inflammatory disease. The watery content of the hydrosalpinx appears white on this T2 signal of MR imaging. The string of beads appearance of hydrosalpinx reflects the luminal structure of the fallopian tube.

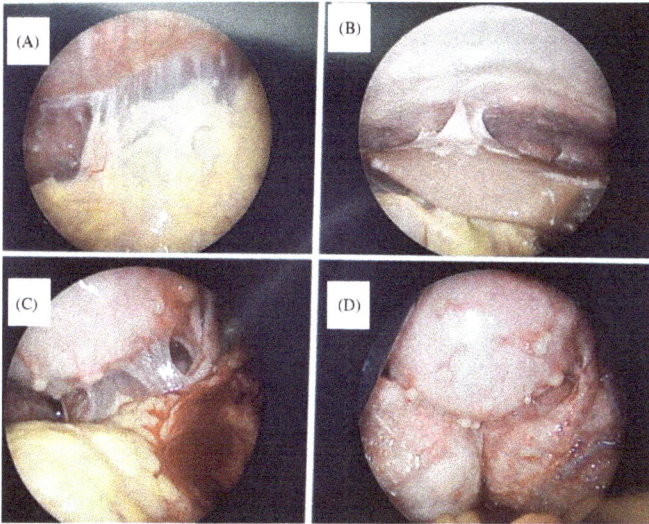

This panel of photographs obtained during investigation of chronic pelvic pain in a 30-year-old woman reveals severe adhesions involving the anterior abdominal wall peritoneum (panel (A)), peri-hepatic space (panel (B)), the Pouch of Douglas (panel (C)) and the gross bilateral hydrosalpinx (panel (D)). This phenomenon is also known as the Fitz-Hugh-Curtis syndrome. In this case, the etiology of the pelvic inflammatory disease was M tuberculosis.

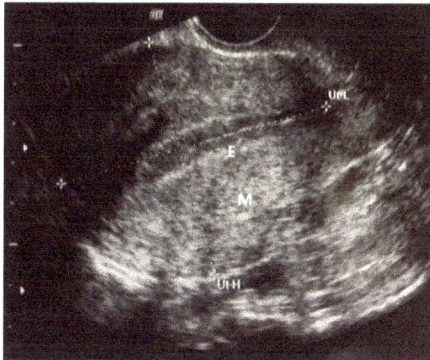

This photograph of an ultrasound scan of the uterus shows the markedly thickened myometrium (marked "M") of the posterior wall of the uterus, typical of adenomyosis. Uterine adenomyosis typically causes dysmenorrhea. In chronic and severe cases, the pain can extend to before and after the actual menstruation to cause chronic pelvic pain.

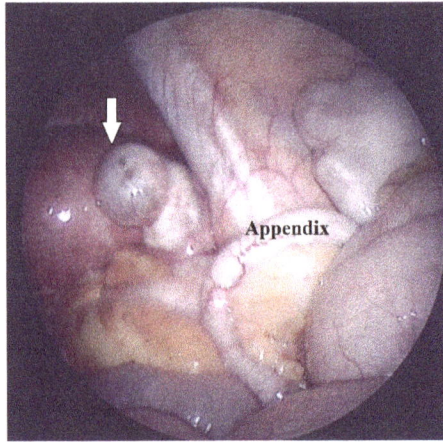

This woman complained of mid-cycle lower abdominal pain. The photograph of a laparoscopy shows the ovulatory follicle (white arrow) on the ovary. The pain associated with ovulation is known as Mittelschmerz which means "middle pain" literally in German. The close proximity of the appendix can cause confusion between Mittelschmerz and acute appendicitis.

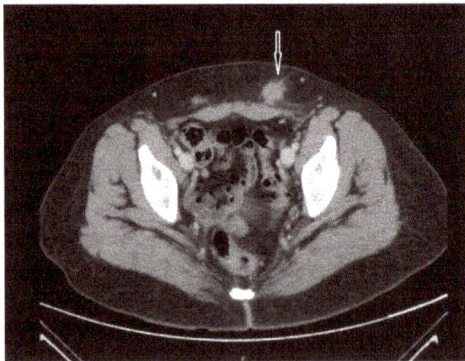

This 35-year-old woman with one child delivered by a lower segment caesarean section 4 years previously complained of a left iliac fossa pain for 3 years. The pain was worse during menstrual period. Examination found a 2-cm nodule beneath the abdominal scar of the caesarean section. This photograph of a CT scan shows a nodule in the subcutaneous compartment of the anterior abdominal wall. It was an endometrioma of the scar, typically a development from seedling of endometrial tissue to the scar during caesarean section. She had not had any pelvic endometriosis.

CASE 19 — ABDOMINAL SWELLING

A 50-year-old woman complains that her abdominal girth is getting bigger over the last four weeks.

- What particular history would be helpful in reaching a diagnosis?
- How does one ascertain that the mass is a pelvic lesion?
- How should this patient be investigated?

What Particular History would be Helpful in Reaching a Diagnosis?

Expansion of abdominal girth may arise from weight gain and obesity, visceral organomegaly, chronic bladder distension, ascites, intra-abdominal tumor or malignancy, pelvic tumor or malignancy, pregnancy in women of reproductive age, and endocrinopathy such as Cushing syndrome.

A history of enhanced appetite and increased food consumption, with or without dietary changes, suggests that the rising abdominal girth may be due to weight gain. The patient may exhibit symptoms and signs of an underlying affective disorder, anxiety state, or psychological stress.

Pregnancy at the end of the spectrum of reproductive age is uncommon but the diagnosis may be dismissed by women who assume that experience of amenorrhea is due to menstrual irregularity preceding menopause. History of nausea and vomiting may either be mild or absent.

Uterine fibroid, the most common tumor in women of reproductive life, can present with an abdominal swelling.

The abdominal distension is usually painless and may be associated with menorrhagia or urinary symptoms, most commonly frequency of micturition and a sensation of incomplete voiding.

Chronic bladder distension is associated with a history of urinary frequency and incontinence of an overflow type. In women, it occurs predominantly in neurogenic conditions such as stroke, paraplegia, multiple sclerosis, and post-surgical neuropathy. It also occurs in a small proportion of women after bladder neck surgery such as urethral sling operation. Very rarely, bladder outlet obstruction is brought on by a large cervical or vaginal tumor.

A massive hepatomegaly presenting with abdominal bloating or enlargement, with or without ascites, is most commonly caused by tumors, either primary or metastatic. History of a malignancy, chronic alcoholism and viral hepatitis carrier status points to the definitive diagnosis.

Large ascites is often associated with lack of appetite and effort intolerance from ventilatory respiration compromise. Enquiry should be made on history of malignancy, liver disease, drug consumption, and intraperitoneal manipulation such as dialysis and drug delivery. A systemic history review of the gastrointestinal tract, urinary tract and reproductive system is crucial for identifying a potential undiagnosed primary malignancy from these organs.

How does one Ascertain that the Mass is a Pelvic Lesion?

Clinical signs revealed on comprehensive physical examination often lead to a probable diagnosis of abdominal distension. Inference of pelvic origin of a mass palpable on abdominal examination is classically described in the phrase "cannot get below it." This is confirmed on bimanual examination of the pelvis from combined abdominal and vaginal approach.

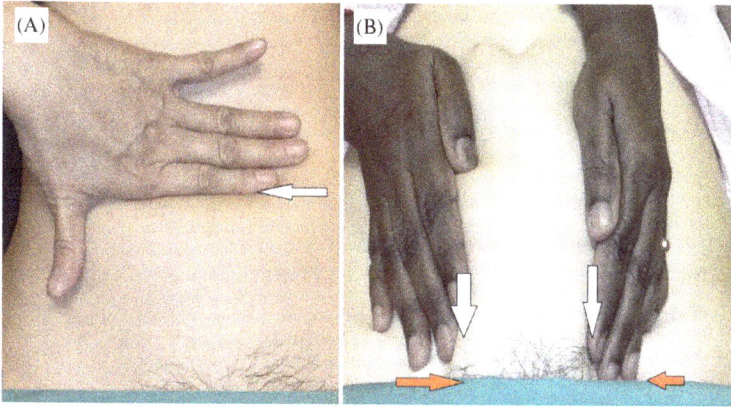

This photographs shows the technique of clinical examination of an abdomino-pelvic mass. Panel (A) shows the upper border of the mass below the radial border of the index finger (marked by the white arrow). In panel (B), the two vertical white arrows mark the lateral borders of the mass extending to the level of pubic rami (marked by two orange color arrows). The pubic rami stop the examination hands from moving further downwards, thus the expression "cannot get below it".

How should this Patient be Investigated?

The primary investigations aim to identify the origin of the pathologic lesion and assess the risk of malignancy.

(i) **Ultrasonography**, the initial investigation of choice, can accurately delineate the origin and tissue consistency of pelvic masses. It distinguishes solid uterine masses from cystic or solid-cystic ovarian masses. It also detects pelvic peritoneal nodules and ascites.

(ii) **MRI** provides invaluable tissue features such as the presence of fluid, fat, mucin, hemorrhage and other soft tissues for further characterization of the mass and is often helpful in distinguishing benign from malignant ovarian masses. It is also highly specific for uterine myometrial masses such as fibroid, adenomyoma and sarcoma. MRI also delineates accurately the depth of myometrial invasion of endometrial tumors. Furthermore, MRI allows assessment of retroperitoneal compartment of the pelvis for ureteric pathology and lymphadenopathy.

(iii) **Serum tumor marker panel**, though not specific, provides invaluable information for risk of malignancy assessment in the presence of a pelvic mass. Epithelial ovarian carcinoma and primary peritoneal carcinoma are often associated with markedly elevated serum CA125 and, less often, a CEA and CA19.9. Ovarian germ cell tumor may be positive for raised serum α-feto-protein (AFP), β-HCG and lactate dehydrogenase.

(iv) **Upper and lower gastrointestinal track endoscopy** is indicated in the presence of dyspeptic symptoms, early satiety, or a history of change of bowel habits. Disseminated primary tumors of gastrointestinal tract commonly involves peritoneum and pelvic organs, particularly the ovaries and manifest as abdominal distension.

Selected Diseases

1. Uterine Fibroids

It is estimated that uterine fibroids occur in 80% of women during the lifespan. The incidence is higher among African women than Caucasians. Other known risk factors for fibroid development are nulliparity, high body mass index, and increasing age.

Uterine fibroid is a benign uterine muscle neoplasm characterized by overgrowth of muscle cells and fibrous tissue. It has a hard consistency, white whirled cut surface, and a pseudo-capsule made up of compressed peripheral muscle layers. Fibroid is monoclonal in cell type and individual fibroids on the same uterus develop separately with different clones, some involving aberrations in chromosomes 6, 7, 12 or 14. There is, however, no Mendelian pattern of inheritance in fibroid development. The growth of fibroids is enhanced by estrogen, progesterone and insulin-like growth factors. The average growth rate is approximately 1-cm per year during premenopausal years, but periods of rapid growth spurts occur, consistence with the biology of benign neoplasm and with no evidence of increased risk of malignant transformation. De novo malignant transformation of fibroid is extremely rare. Uterine sarcoma is found in no more than 0.2% of hysterectomy done for uterine fibroids. During the postmenopausal years, when estrogen replacement therapy is not instituted, some but not all, fibroids show gradual and substantial regression, but never completely disappear.

Fibroids are clinically described by their location in relation to uterine serosa, myometrium and endometrium as submucous, intramural and subserosal. In the FIGO classification of abnormal uterine bleeding, uterine fibroids are classified into nine types:

• *Submucous: 3 types*

Type-0: intracavitary fibroid polyp with a narrow stalk
Type-1: <50% of fibroid mass involving uterine myometrium
Type-2: ≥50% of fibroid mass involving the myometrium

• *Intramural: 2 types*

Type-3: intramural fibroid abutting endometrium
Type-4: fibroid not abutting endometrium and serosa

• *Subserosal: 3 types*

Type-5: ≥50% extension of the mass into myometrium
Type-6: <50% extension of the mass into myometrium
Type-7: fibroid connected to the serosa with a narrow stalk (pedunculated)

• *Fibroids not involving myometrium*

Type-8: cervical fibroids, broad ligament fibroids, round ligament fibroids and parasitic fibroids.

Most fibroids (>60%) are asymptomatic. The most common symptom, if present, is abnormal uterine bleeding which includes heavy menstrual bleeding, prolonged uterine bleeding, and intermenstrual bleeding. This is generally a complication of submucosal fibroids. Other fibroids are associated with mass compression symptoms such as abdominal distension, bladder dysfunction, including urinary frequency, sensation of incomplete voiding, or acute retention of urine, bower dysfunction including constipation, and rarely vascular compression with venous stasis of the lower limbs and deep vein thrombosis. Fibroids may be a cause of infertility and a risk factor for miscarriage. Fibroids can undergo avascular necrosis or degeneration causing abdominal pain. Hemorrhage into the necrotic tissue causes a beefy consistency or red degeneration more often, but not exclusively, encountered during pregnancy.

The diagnosis of fibroid is presumed for a firm and irregular lower abdominal mass arising out of the pelvis, or the uterus is found to be enlarged, firm in consistency and irregular in contour on bimanual examination of the pelvis. Pelvic ultrasound scan is the investigation of the first choice as it reliably distinguishes ovarian mass, pregnancy, hematometra, or uterine adenomyosis and adenomyoma as the cause a large pelvic mass. The salient ultrasnographic feature of an uncomplicated fibroid appears hypoechoic as compared with normal myometrium. Fibroids can be calcified. Degenerative fibroids may show cystic areas of necrosis. Complex ultrasound features of mixed echogenicity with increased blood flow patterns on Doppler study may raise a suspicion, but not diagnostic, of a uterine sarcoma. An endometrial stromal sarcoma may be indistinguishable from a submucous fibroid.

Uncommonly, a complex case may be investigated with a pelvic MRI. MRI distinguishes a pedunculated fibroid from an adnexal mass. Typically, an uncomplicated fibroid appears as a focal mass of low to intermediate T1 signal intensity and low T2 signal intensity on MRI. High signal intensity is seen in degenerative or cystic areas of fibroids. A uterine mass of irregular contour with mixed low and high signal intensity may suggest, but again not diagnostic, of a leiomyosarcoma.

Heavy uterine bleeding in the presence of a fibroid should be investigated for other possible causes such as thyroid dysfunction, von Willebrand's disease and coagulopathy (if heavy bleeding dates back to menarche), and uterine hyperplasia or carcinoma.

The majority of fibroids do not require treatment. Choice of treatment of symptomatic fibroid is a woman's autonomous decision taking into consideration the severity and type of symptoms, wish for and plan of fertility, and acceptability of medications or surgery.

(i) *Expectant management*

Asymptomatic fibroids resulting in a uterine enlargement to a gestation size of less than 12 weeks can be managed expectantly. These women should be instructed on seeking prompt medical attention on development of abnormal uterine bleeding, abdominal pain or increasing abdominal distention. Yearly ultrasound scan to monitor the dimension of the fibroid is unnecessary as the findings are not predictive of growth of the fibroid. Women planning for pregnancy within the following 12 months should undergo an initial investigation for factors of subfertility and re-evaluated if pregnancy does not occur during the ensuing six months.

(ii) *Medical therapy*

Medical therapy aims to control symptoms, particularly heavy uterine bleeding. It is not a curative treatment of fibroids.

- Tranexamic acid, an anti-fibrinolytic agent, given at 1000 mg trice daily during menstruation, has been established as the first-line medical therapy for these women. As the treatment duration is limited to a few days during menstruation, the treatment is well tolerated and carries a minimum risk of adverse reactions.
- Combined oral contraceptive pills and intrauterine levonorgestrel delivery system (Mirena) are the alternative therapies with additional benefit on dysmenorrhea.

- Non-steroidal anti-inflammatory agents have also been used to achieve a mild to moderate reduction in menstrual bleeding and dysmenorrhea.
- Low dose danazol at 200 mg daily also significantly reduces menstrual blood loss. However, androgenic side effects make it intolerable for long-term use.
- Aromatase inhibitors: limited available data have reported the efficacy of these agents on reducing menstrual bleeding.
- Progesterone-receptor modulating agents: Mifepristone for medical termination of early pregnancy and ulipristal acetate for emergency contraception following unprotected sexual intercourse or contraceptive failure have been reported to reduce heavy menstrual bleeding and fibroid volume. Oral administration of ulipristal acetate 5 mg to 10 mg daily for four months have been shown to result in reduced heavy menstrual bleeding or amenorrhea and a reduction of uterine volume by 40%. The benefits are sustained for up to six months duration. The four-month course of treatment can be repeated when necessary but clinical experience and safety of long-term intermittent treatment are lacking. The most common adverse effects reported are hot flushes, headaches, abdominal pain, fatigue, weight gaining, breast pain, and acne.
- GnRH analogues, by suppressing ovarian functions, induce a reversible state of amenorrhea and shrinkage of the fibroid. This line of therapy is effective in treating heavy menstrual bleeding and compressive symptoms from the bulk of the fibroid. Short-term treatment with GnRH analogues is widely employed in women before myomectomy and when a woman is near menopause. The treatment is significantly associated with estrogen deficiency syndrome and bone loss. In young women, cessation of GnRH analogue treatment is associated with re-growth of the fibroid to pre-treatment size within the following six months.

(iii) *Uterine artery embolization (UAE) therapy*

Embolization of uterine arteries with polyvinyl alcohol (PVA) or pingyangmycin lipiodol emulsion and silk-segment (PLES) are established minimally invasive treatment of symptomatic fibroids with conservation of the uterus. It is a choice for women who declines or are unfit for surgery. Compared to myomectomy, UAE carries a similar efficacy in symptomatic improvement but has a shorter hospitalization stay and earlier return to normal daily activities and work. On the other hand, UAE has a higher reported rate of short-term minor complications and hospital re-admission, and surgical re-intervention within five years. Limited data also suggest that myomectomy is preferred to UAE for fertility outcome. Technical failure of UAE is reported in 5% to 10% of patients.

(iv) *MRI-guided focused ultrasound surgery*

Real-time MR imaging of the fibroids allows noninvasive delivery of high intensity focused ultrasound energy to the targeted tissue for thermal ablation. Gradual reduction of the volume of fibroid ensues and a total volume reduction of 30% at three-year follow-up has been reported. The outcome on long-term follow up is yet to be seen.

(v) *Hysteroscopic myomectomy*

This is a minimally invasive curative treatment of fibroids and the fibroid tissues are available for histological assessment and diagnosis. Fibroid polyps, submucosal fibroids and intramural fibroids encroaching on the endometrial cavity (FIGO types 0–4) are potential candidates for transcervical hysteroscopic resection surgery. The surgical duration and success of complete resection of the fibroids are related to the size of the fibroid, its location in the uterus and its extent within the uterine myometrium. Fibroids of more than 5 cm in diameter and deep myometrial extension of two thirds or more of the full myometrial thickness, in particular those located in the upper one third or the lateral wall of the uterus, are best treated by alternative surgical methods.

The short-term success rate for menstrual bleeding control is achieved in 70% to 90% of patients after hysteroscopic resection of fibroids. The rate is higher with concomitant endometrial ablation in women who have completed fertility. The failure rate increases with the duration of follow up because of recurrence of fibroids and development of other causes of heavy menstrual bleeding. Improved fertility rate after this procedure is notable in types 0–2 fibroids. The procedure is safe but surgical complications include uterine perforation, cervical trauma, fluid overload and electrolyte imbalance, and intrauterine adhesions.

(vi) Abdominal myomectomy

Laparoscopic and laparotomy myomectomy are effective methods of curative treatment of subserosal and intramural fibroids. Laparoscopic myomectomy is preferred to laparotomy for its shorter recovery duration. However, laparoscopic myomectomy requires intra-abdominal power morcellation, a technique associated with a risk of dissemination of tumor cells in inadvertent treatment of a leiomyosarcoma.

Abdominal myomectomy carries a significant rate of surgical complications which include conversion to hysterectomy, infertility from adhesion formation, and uterine rupture during pregnancy and labor. Almost 25% of women require subsequent treatment for recurrence of fibroids.

(vii) *Hysterectomy*

Hysterectomy accounts for three quarters of surgeries for fibroids. It is a permanent cure of fibroids and a definitive treatment of concurrent uterine diseases such as adenomyosis, abnormal uterine bleeding, and cervical neoplasia. There is a high satisfaction rate of hysterectomy with a marked improvement in quality of life at 10-year follow up, despite a significant surgical morbidity during operation and the early postoperative period.

Hysterectomy is a suitable option for women who have completed childbearing. Where the size of the fibroid allows, vaginal hysterectomy or laparoscopy assisted vaginal hysterectomy is the surgical method of choice for its low complication rate. In abdominal approach of hysterectomy, minimally invasive laparoscopy or laparoscopy assisted robotic procedure is preferred to laparotomy for its shorter postoperative recovery time and less pain. The minimally invasive surgery requires power morcellation of the organ for its removal. The procedure carries a risk of inadvertent tumor dissemination in cases of undiagnosed uterine cancer.

2. Ovarian Cancer

In Singapore, ovarian cancer ranked fifth in the most common cancers and accounted for 5.5% of all cancers in women between 2010 and 2014. The age standardized incidence is 12.8 per 100,000 women. In contrast to a recent decline in the number of cases in the USA, ovarian cancer in Singapore has been on a steadily rising trend over the last 40 years. Ovarian cancer can occur in women of all age groups but the proportion distribution of the cases is approximately 25% in women below 45-years old, 55% in women between 45 and 64-years old, and 20% in women aged 65-years or older.

Ovaries are common sites of metastatic cancers from the colon, stomach and breasts. Appropriate investigation is needed to exclude a primary cancer elsewhere before coming to a diagnosis of a primary ovarian cancer. Almost 90% of all primary ovarian

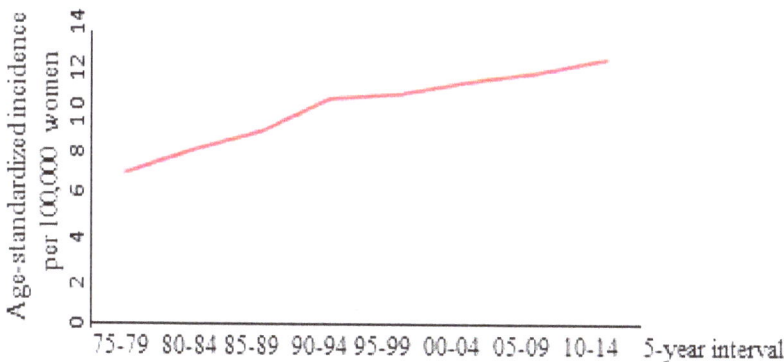

This chart illustrates the rising incidence trend in ovarian cancer in Singapore between 1975 and 2014.

cancers are epithelial in origin. The remaining 10% of ovarian cancers arise from germ cells, sex cord and, rarely, from other cell types.

Epithelial ovarian cancer arises from surface epithelium which is coelomic in its embryonic origin, in common with Müllerian tube development. Histologically, epithelial ovarian cancer can assume the lineage of Müllerian differentiation to become serous, endometrioid, mucinous and clear cell carcinoma. Recent evidence indicates that high-grade serous carcinoma of the ovary has an origin in fimbrial epithelium of the fallopian tube. Endometrioid and clear cell carcinoma may be arising from endometriosis.

Approximately 20% of epithelial ovarian cancers are classified into a separate entity of borderline ovarian tumor (BOT) which carries an excellent prognosis. Meticulous pathological examination is required for a diagnosis of BOT. Importantly, the number of mitosis is less than 4 per 10 high-power field, nuclear atypia and increase in nuclear/cytoplasmic ratio are mild, and tissue architecture shows epithelial multi-layering of not more than 4 cell layers, branching of epithelial papillae and pseudopapillae is slight, and destructive stromal invasion must be absent.

Malignant germ cell tumors occur in young women. The most common types are immature teratoma and dysgerminoma. Yolk sac tumor, embryonal tumor and choriocarcinoma are rare. There are also mixed tumors of more than one cell type. Immature teratoma composes of embryonal tissues from ectoderm, mesoderm and endoderm. All dysgerminoma are considered malignant but only one third of the cases behave aggressively. About 5% of dysgerminoma occur in dysgenesis of the gonads.

Epidemiological evidence demonstrates a higher risk for epithelial ovarian cancer in nulliparous as compared with multiparous women and a lower risk among women who have ever used combined estrogen-progestogen birth control pills. It is believed that incessant ovulations play an important etiological role in development of epithelial ovarian cancer as the frequent tissue repair following ovulation increases the probability of aberrant cellular proliferation. Mutation in p53 oncogene is found in almost all cases of high-grade serous carcinoma and a number of other genetic aberrations have been identified in other types of epithelial ovarian cancer. The overall background risk of epithelial ovarian cancer is estimated to be 1.6% in women with no family history of ovarian cancer. This risk increases for women whose first-degree family members have history of ovarian cancer: 4% for one member and 7% for two or more members. Less than 10% of ovarian cancer women come from specific genetic syndromes of BRCA1 and BRCA2 family or Lynch syndrome with altered mismatch repair genes.

Ovarian cancer spread by direct local invasion of pelvic visceral, transcoelomically to involve pelvic and abdominal peritoneum, abdominal visceral and omentum, and transdiaphramatically to thoracic space and pleural membranes. Lymphatic infiltration leading to pelvic and para-aorto-caval lymph nodes is common but hematogenous metastasis to liver, lungs or distant locations occurs predominantly only in advanced cancer.

Ovarian cancer is a silent disease in the early stage. Disease at a more advanced stage may present with vague symptoms of abdominal bloating, early satiety and loss of appetite and body weight, constipation, urinary frequency, lower limb edema or breathlessness. Some patients feel an abdominal mass. Physical examination may detect an abdominal-pelvic mass, ascites and/or pleural effusion.

The objectives of investigation of ovarian cancer are: (1) confirming the primary origin of ovarian tumor; (2) evaluating the risk of malignant nature of the tumor; and (3) assessing the extent of the tumor. Ultrasound scan is sensitive for confirming the ovarian location of the tumor but endoscopy may be warranted in suitable patients to exclude a gastrointestinal cancer and a mammography may detect a breast malignancy. The International Ovarian Tumor Analysis (IOTA) group has established ultrasound scan rules for benign and malignant tumors with a 95% sensitivity and 91% specificity. The IOTA's "M" rule for malignancy include:

- Irregular solid tumor, tumor with four or more papillary structures
- Irregular multilocular tumor nodules of 10 cm or more in diameter

- Tumor with very high blood flow
- Presence of ascites.

Serum CA125 level is elevated in 80% of epithelial ovarian cancer in general but, on its own, has low sensitivity and specificity. A risk of malignancy index (RMI) calculated by combining ultrasound scan findings, serum CA125 level and menopausal status has been established since 1990 as below:

RMI = U × M × CA125

Where U is the ultrasound score. 1 point is assigned to each of the following characteristics: multilocular cysts, solid areas, metastases, ascites and bilateral lesions. U = 0 (for an ultrasound score of 0), U = 1 (for an ultrasound score of 1), U = 3 (for an ultrasound score of 2–5).

M is the menopausal status (premenopausal = 1 and postmenopausal = 3).

Serum CA-125 is the absolute measurement in IU/mL.

The pooled data from 36 studies in a systemic review showed that an RMI score of 200 has a sensitivity of 78% (95% CI 71–85%) and specificity of 87% (95% CI 83–91%) for the detection of ovarian malignancies. This assessment is useful for identifying patients in whom the ovarian masses are at high risk of malignancy and who should best be managed by gynecologic oncologists.

In young women whose ovarian tumors may be germ cell in origin, assessment of serum tumor markers should include β-HCG, α-fetoprotein, and lactate dehydrogenase.

CT-scan of the thorax, abdomen and pelvis provides an overall assessment of the extent of tumor involvement in these regions. MRI, by its ability to characterize tissue types: hemorrhage, fat, mucin and serous fluid has an additional advantage of identifying benign nature of the tumor.

Diagnosis of malignancy may be confirmed on cytological examination of aspirate samples from pleural fluid or ascites or on histological assessment of fine needle biopsies of the tumor. Approximately 10% of cases thus diagnosed are proven to be wrong in subsequent laparotomy diagnosis. These techniques also cause significant delay in the definitive treatment of ovarian cancer and are not to be recommended as a routine procedure. They may be used in women with poor health where a laparotomy carries an unacceptable risk.

Laparotomy is the standard of care for surgical management of primary epithelial ovarian cancer. The staging procedure involves aspiration of ascitic fluid or obtaining peritoneal washing for cytology, careful inspection of the ovarian tumor and pelvic condition, meticulous exploratory examination of peritoneum, abdominal visceral, diaphragm and retroperitoneal structures in the pelvis and para-aorto-caval spaces. Representative biopsies are obtained. Debulking surgery is performed with an aim to optimally cytoreduce the tumor. Complete cytoreduction with total hysterectomy, bilateral salpingo-oophorectomy, omentectomy and retroperitoneal lymph node dissection, and sometimes visceral resection where necessary, is the best desirable outcome. Tumor excision to an extent that the residual tumor is less than 1-cm in the greatest diameter is considered an optimal cytoreduction.

Laparoscopic surgery is limited to diagnostic purpose. It may also be used to treat a stage IA ovarian cancer. Fertility sparing surgery in young women with stage IA cancer and for women with germ cell tumors is achieved by conserving the contralateral ovary and the uterus after the staging exploration.

In surgically unfit patients and in patients with extensive tumor, where optimal cytoreductive surgery is deemed impossible, neo-adjuvant chemotherapy is recommended with a plan to perform an interval debulking surgery after three cycles of chemotherapy. This approach improves the probability of subsequent optimal surgery and reduces perioperative morbidity.

With the exception of FIGO stage 1A grade-1 carcinoma, all cases of ovarian cancer are treated with combined taxane-carboplatin chemotherapy for six cycles.

Primary ovarian cancer is staged using FIGO staging classification. Stage 1 refers to tumor confined to one or both ovaries. Stage 2 refers to tumor extending to structures confined to the true pelvis. Stage 3 refers to tumor involving the abdominal cavity or retroperitoneal lymph nodes. Stage 4 refers to distant metastasis and parenchymal metastasis of the liver and spleen.

Prognosis of ovarian cancer is related to the FIGO stage of the disease, degree of cytoreductive surgery and response to chemotherapy. The 5-year survival rate is 90% for stage 1, 70% for stage 2, 50% for stage 3 and 10% for stage 4. The overall 5-year survival rate is 45%. Ovarian cancer is the commonest cause of mortality in all gynecological cancers. On the other hand, borderline ovarian tumor has a 10-year mortality rate of less than 5% and germ cell tumors are curable cancers.

Routine screening for ovarian cancer in the general population is not recommended for three reasons: low population prevalence of the disease, lack of precancerous stage for intervention to prevent cancer, and lack of a reliable specific screening test. Routine annual transvaginal ultrasound scan of the ovaries in high-risk population and serial serum CA125 assays for a rising trend in postmenopausal women may allow detection of ovarian cancer in an early stage.

Illustration of Some Conditions that Present with Abdominal Swellings

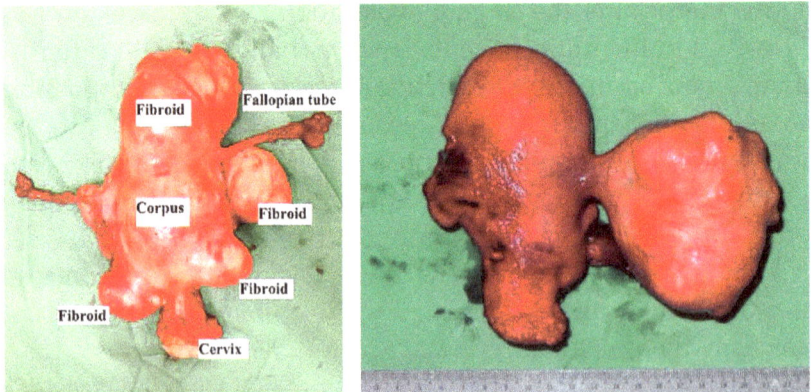

These photographs show the specimens from total hysterectomies. The distorted contour from multiple fibroids in the left panel, and by a large pedunculated fibroid (right panel) contributes to the findings on clinical examination of the uterus.

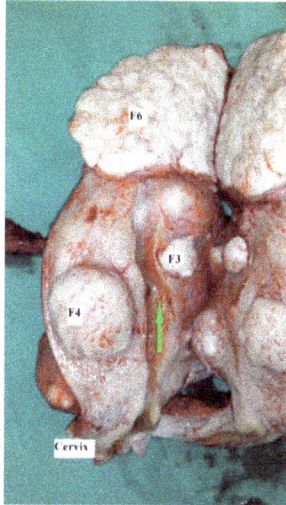

This photograph shows the cut specimen of a hysterectomy. There were multiple fibroids. The green arrow points to the endometrial cavity. F3 and F4 are the FIGO type-3 and type-4 intramural fibroids, and F6 is the FIGO type-6 subserosal fibroid. F6 also demonstrates the typical whitish dense fibrous cut surface with whirl appearance of a fibroid.

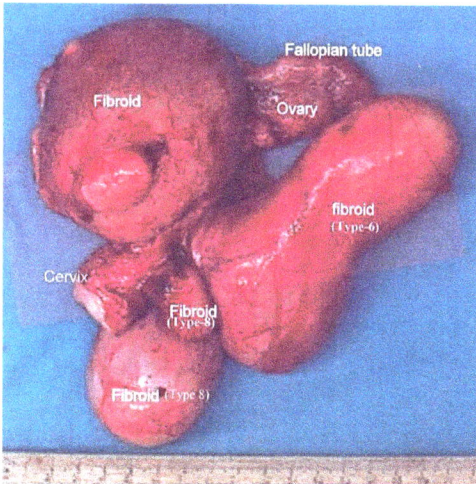

This photograph shows a total hysterectomy specimen. There were multiple fibroids in the corpus and the cervix (FIGO type-8) and subserosal fibroid with <50% myometrial extension (FIGO type-6).

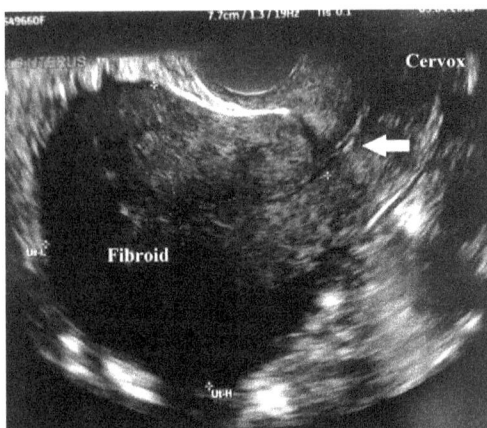

This photograph of an ultrasound image of the longitudinal section of the uterus shows a large fibroid at the fundus of the uterus. It shows the typical hypoechoic feature of ultrasound scan. The white arrow points to the endometrial cavity.

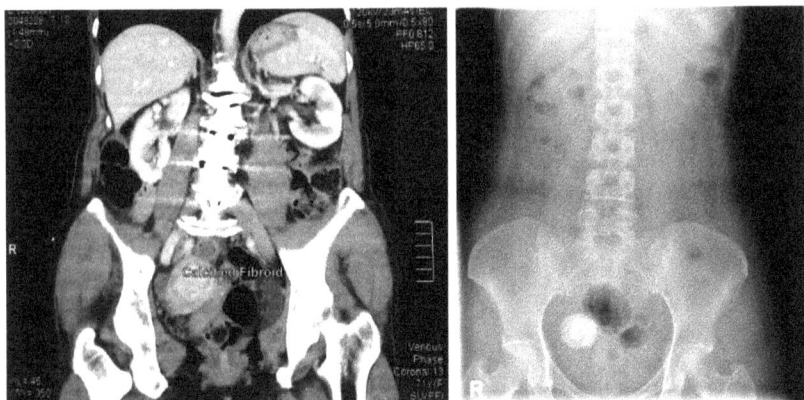

These photographs show a coronal section of a CT-KUB image (left panel) and a plain abdominal X-ray (right panel). The radio opaque lesion in the pelvis is a calcified fibroid.

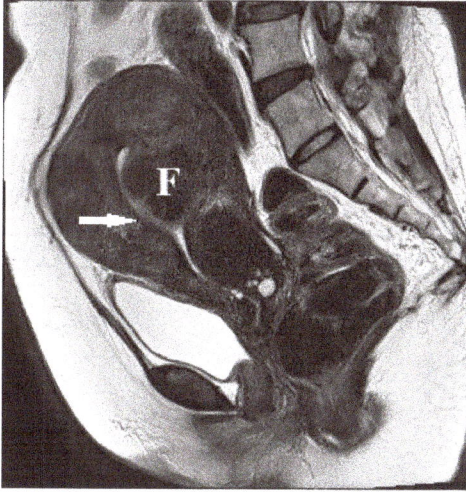

This photograph of a MR image (T2 Signal) shows a fibroid (marked "F") extending into the endometrial cavity (white arrow).

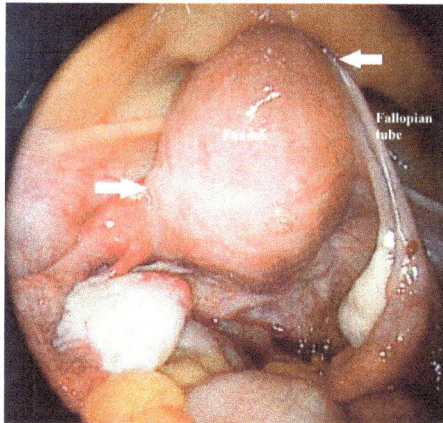

This photograph of a laparoscopy shows that the uterus was grossly enlarged. The fundus of the uterus was elevated as shown by the asymmetry in the level of the uterine-fallopian tube junctions between the right and left hand sides (marked by the white arrows). There was a large subserosal fibroid.

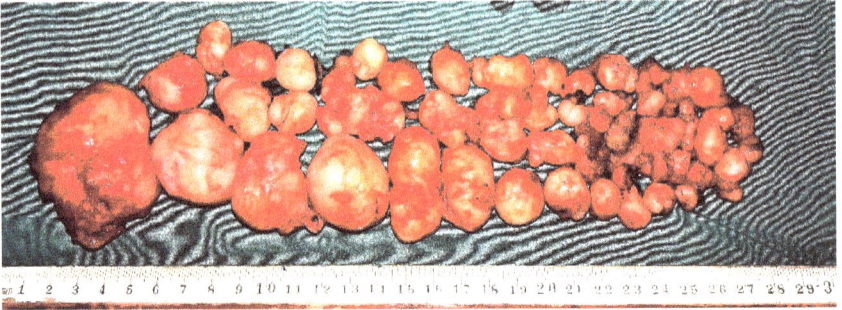

This photograph shows 51 fibroids removed from the uterus of a young woman who desired fertility.

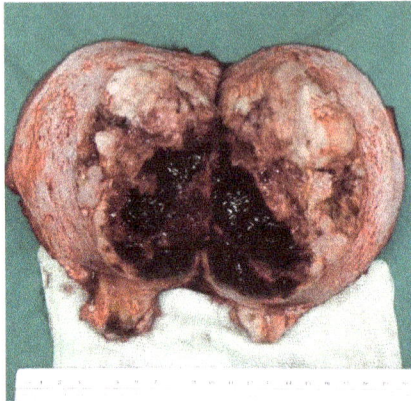

This 55-year-old postmenopausal woman complained of a dull ache in the lower abdomen. She was found to have an enlarged uterus to a 12-week gestational size. The uterus was tender. An ultrasound scan showed a large intramural fibroid with cystic spaces. The differential diagnosis included a degenerated fibroid and leiomyosarcoma. The cut specimen of the total hysterectomy revealed a large hemorrhagic tumor with necrosis in the myometrium. Histopathology confirmed a high-grade leiomyosarcoma.

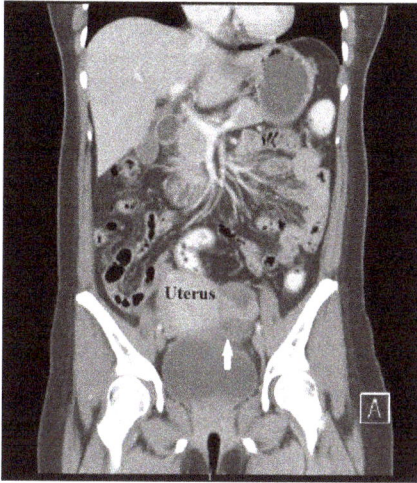

This photograph shows a section of a CT scan which demonstrates a fibroid with cystic degeneration (white arrow).

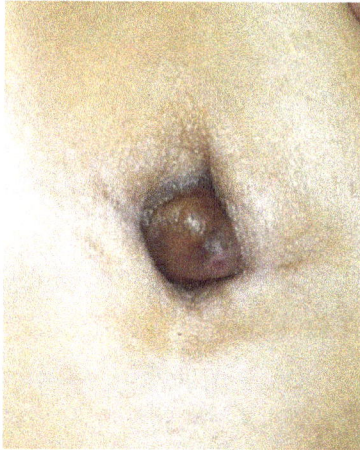

This 40-year-old woman complained of a lump in the abdomen. It was tender and the pain was worse during menstruation. She also had severe dysmenorrhea. The lump was confirmed to be a nodule in the umbilicus. It was an endometriotic nodule.

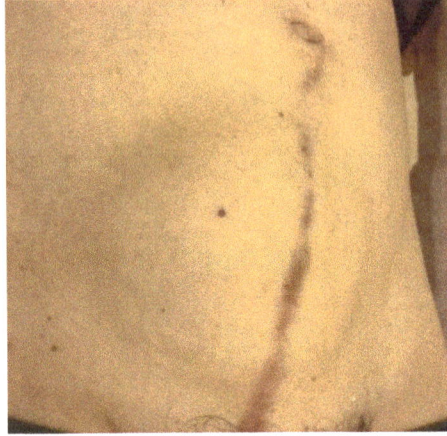

This woman's complaint of an abdominal swelling was a large incisional abdominal hernia from a midline incision for a laparotomy previously.

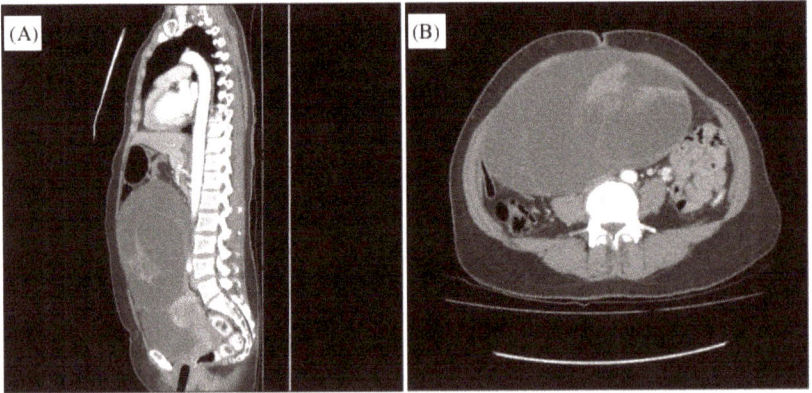

This panel of photographs of CT-scan images showed a huge ovarian tumor. It was a complex tumor with septation and solid areas. This was a mucinous ovarian cancer on histopathology.

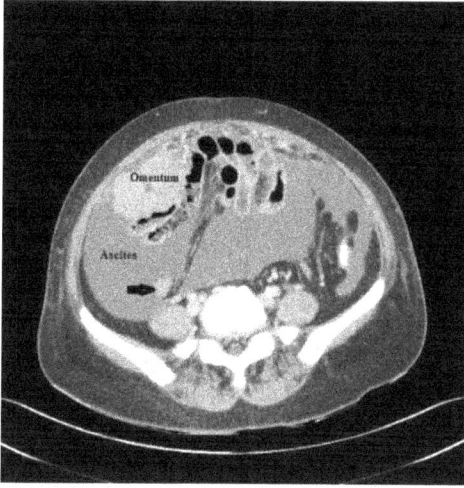

This patient had a hugely distended abdomen from tense ascites. The photograph shows a section of CT scan demonstrating huge ascites, omental caking and peritoneal tumor deposits (black arrow) from advanced ovarian carcinoma.

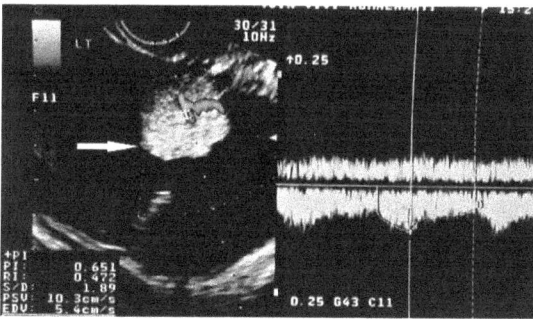

This photograph of an image from ultrasound scan shows an ovarian tumor (marked by arrow) and the increased blood flow pattern on Doppler study.

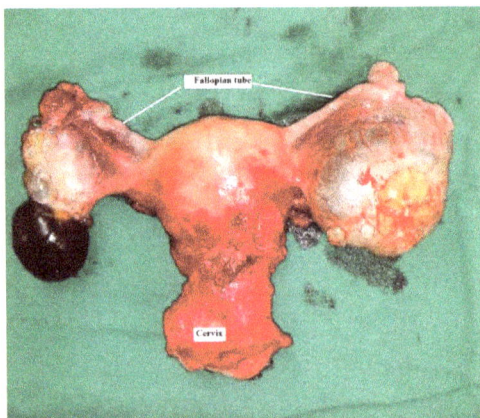

This photograph shows a surgical specimen of total hysterectomy and bilateral salpingo-oophorectomy. The ovarian tumors were recognizable by the ovarian capsular tumor excrescences.

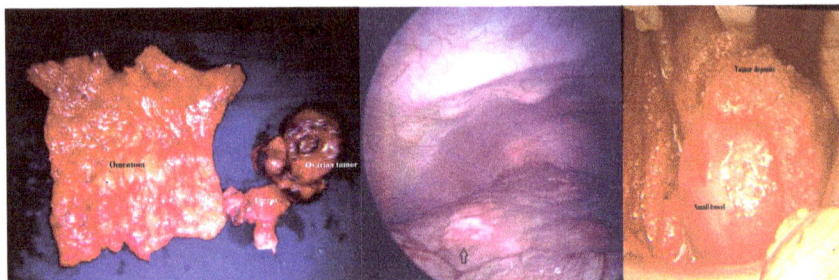

This photographs shows the laparotomy staging of an ovarian cancer. The procedure includes total hysterectomy, bilateral salpingo-oophorectomy, omentectomy (panel on the left), bowel and other abdominal visceral survey (liver metastasis shown in the middle panel and marked by open arrow) and resection, and retroperitoneal lymphadenectomy (not shown on this photographs).

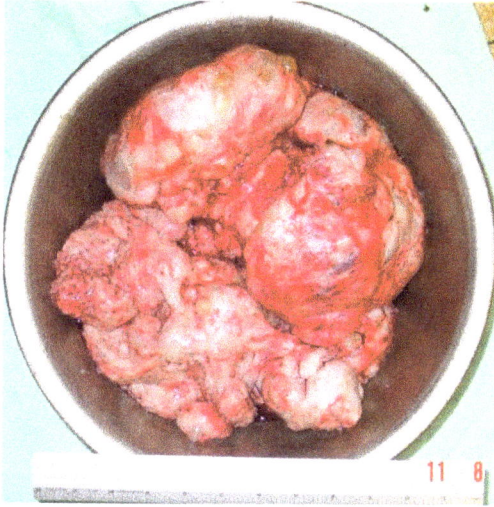

This 20-year-old woman had a huge right ovarian immature teratoma which filled the entire basin of 30 cm in diameter. She undertook right salpingo-oophorectomy and received chemotherapy and had been disease free for the 5-year follow up. She had also resumed normal menstruation.

CASE 20 — CERVICAL SCREENING

A 30-year-old woman requests to be screened for cervical cancer.

- What are the objectives of cervical screening?
- What validated screening tests are available?
- How to manage abnormal screening results?
- What is the primary prevention method of cervical cancer?

What are the Objectives of Cervical Screening?

Cervical cancer screening is the first established population screening for cancer in medical history. Cervical cancer is high in prevalence and in morbidity and mortality. Early invasive cervical cancer has a relatively long asymptomatic phase amenable to curative treatment. More importantly, squamous cell carcinoma, the most common type of cervical cancer, is preceded by a decade-long pre-invasive cervical intraepithelial neoplasia (CIN). Treatment of CIN effectively prevents subsequent development of invasive cervical carcinoma. While tumor biology is favorable, cervical cancer screening is possible only because of available sensitive and specific diagnostic tests for pre-invasive and invasive disease. The objectives of cervical cancer screening, therefore, are: (i) to detect early cervical cancer for early treatment to reduce the morbidity and mortality from the cancer and to improve quality of life of these women; and (ii) to detect high-grade CIN for appropriate treatment to prevent development of invasive cervical cancer.

What Validated Screening Tests are Available?

(i) Cervical Cytology Test

Works on exfoliated cervical cytology started 100 years ago and Dr George Papanicolaou published the use of cytology in the detection of cervical cancer in 1923. The name of "Pap-smear" has since been attached to the test. The conventional cytology involves smearing a sample of cervical scrape directly onto a microscopy glass slide for staining and microscopic examination. The liquid-based cytology (LBC) involves washing the sample cells into a cell preservation solution. The sample is processed and cells are prepared in monolayer for staining and microscopic examination.

Experience in cervical cancer mass screening over the last 50 years has established that the sensitivity and specificity of cytology test for CIN3 is 70% and 90%, respectively. The sensitivity of screening can be improved with regular screening at three-yearly interval. As the most at risk population for cervical cancer is women aged between 35-years old and 55-years old and CIN precedes invasive cancer by 10 years, women within this age range are the target for screening. Organized cervical cancer screening program across the globe varies with the age of women entering and exiting the program. In Singapore, the national screening program targets women, who have had sexual intercourse, between the ages of 25-years and 69-years. The test is repeated at three-yearly intervals. Optimal impact of regular screening is seen with more than 80% decrease in the incidence and mortality rate of cervical cancer. This is achieved when 80% or more of the targeted women participate the screening.

(ii) HPV DNA Test

Of the 40 subtypes of human papillomavirus (HPV) that can be found in the anogenital tracts in females, 13 are known to be oncogenic. They are known as high-risk HPV. HPV is a necessary agent in the development of cervical cancer and CIN. Its presence in cervical tissue can be detected with HPV DNA test using polymerase chain reaction technology. The prevalence of high-risk HPV infection is approximately 10% among adult, sexually active women. For the purpose of screening for cervical cancer and CIN3, HPV DNA test has to be adjusted to reflect the presence of the disease rather than the mere presence of HPV. Currently, the only HPV DNA test approved for primary screening purpose is the Cobas 4800 system manufactured by Roche Company (USA).

In a single round of screening, HPV DNA test detected 30% more CIN3 than cytology alone. The early detection of these additional CIN3 cases prevents some cases of invasive cancer that would occur during the interval between successive rounds of screening. This advantage has led some screening program to replace cytology with HPV DNA test as the primary screening method.

Women tested negative for HPV are at extremely low risk of cervical cancer in the ensuing 10 years. This high negative predictive value of the test allows women to lengthen the interval between screens from three years to five to seven years, and to exit screening earlier at 55–60 years old.

(iii) Visual Inspection with Acetic Acid (VIA)

While a tumor on the cervix is recognizable to naked eyes, CIN3 is not. However, both the tumor and CIN of all grades display a whitened appearance after application of 5% acetic acid to the cervix. This has been adopted by low resource countries as the screening test for cervical cancer and CIN3.

The sensitivity and specificity of VIA are approximately 80%, respectively, for the detection of cervical cancer and CIN3. The relatively low specificity has resulted in many women being treated unnecessarily. The optimal interval between VIA screens for optimal cancer screening is unknown.

How to Manage Abnormal Screening Results?

Management of abnormal screening test results depends on the types of test used.

(i) Cytology

Cytology evaluation and findings are reported according to the Bethesda system in two tiers. Based on adequacy of the sample cells and the presence of endocervical and squamous metaplastic cells, the cytology evaluation is classified into two categories, satisfactory and unsatisfactory. Women whose cytology samples are unsatisfactory should undertake a repeat test with a new sample.

Findings on technically satisfactory cytology samples are reported as:

- Negative for intraepithelial lesion or malignancy (NILM) which indicates a normal cervix.
- Low-grade squamous intraepithelial lesions (LSIL): report of this category indicates the presence of abnormal squamous cells ranging from cytopathic effects of HPV infection (koilocytosis) to intraepithelial neoplasia grade-1 (CIN1).
- High-grade squamous intraepithelial lesions (HSIL): report of this category indicates detection of cells arising from severe squamous cell abnormalities ranging from intraepithelial neoplasia grade-2 (CIN2) and grade-3 (CIN3) to invasive cancer.
- Malignant cells present: this indicates detection of cancerous cells. If possible, squamous cell or adenocarcinoma cell type will be stated.
- Atypical squamous cells-undetermined significance (ASCUS): this category includes all squamous epithelial cellular abnormalities that cannot be confidently assigned into one of the above categories. If a likelihood of a high-grade lesion is suspected, it will be assigned as ASC-H or ASCUS favoring high-grade lesions.

- Adenocarcinoma *in situ*: this category denotes neoplastic cells with features of neoplastic glandular abnormality without frank adenocarcinoma.

Management of abnormal cytology results

- Malignant cells present: the patient is referred to a gynecologic oncology clinic for immediate investigation. If a tumor is obvious on naked eye examination, a biopsy is taken for histo-pathology evaluation and diagnosis.

  If no apparent tumor is detected on clinical examination, the cervix is evaluated with colposcopy. A diagnostic biopsy can be performed from the tumorous area. If the colposcopy examination is uncertain of a cancer, a diagnostic cone biopsy should be performed for accurate and reliable diagnosis.
- HSIL: the patient should be referred to a colposcopy clinic within four weeks for evaluation of the cervix. Biopsies are taken from abnormal epithelial lesions for histologic diagnosis. Definitive treatment with local ablative procedure or with an excisional procedure (Loop Electro-Excision Procedure — LEEP, or cone biopsy) will be determined.
- LSIL: the risk of cervical cancer in this category is very low and the cytological abnormalities are largely HPV effects which has a very high spontaneous regression rate (>70%). Women in this category can be observed with a repeat cytology in six months and managed according to the subsequent cytology findings.
- ASCUS: women whose abnormal cytology assigned ASC-H should be referred to a colposcopist for further evaluation.

  The management of the other group of women in the ASCUS category should include a high-risk HPV DNA test. For the group tested positive, they should be referred for colposcopy. Other women can be managed with a repeat cytology test in 12 months.

(ii) HPV DNA Test

Of the 13 HPV subtypes, HPV-16 alone accounts for 50% of CIN and 40–50% of invasive cancer. Collectively HPV-16 and HPV-18 account for 70% of cervical cancer. Among women tested positive for HPV-16 and a normal cytology test, 10% are found to have CIN3.

Management of HPV DNA test on Cobas 4800 system is managed as below:

- HPV-16 and/or HPV-18 positive: These women should be referred for colposcopy within four weeks.
- Other high-risk HPV positive: They should undertake a cytology test. When cytology test is found to be abnormal, the women are evaluated with colposcopy. If cytology is negative, the risk of an existing CIN3/cancer is very low. They can be managed with a repeat HPV DNA test in 12 months.

What is the Primary Prevention Method of Cervical Cancer?

Screening and treatment of CIN3 will interrupt the progressive pathogenesis pathway in the development of cervical cancer. This is known as secondary prevention of cervical cancer. Prevention of oncogenic process by protecting a woman from HPV infection is known as the primary prevention of cervical cancer.

Three HPV vaccines are available:

(i) Cervarix

This is a bivalent vaccine targeting HPV-16 and HPV-18. The vaccine formulation contains an adjuvant substance known as ASO4 (a compound consisting of aluminum hydroxide and monophosphoryl lipid A) which stimulates a stronger and broader immune response to vaccine antigens as compared with adjuvant with aluminum hydroxide alone. This has resulted in cross protection of the vaccine against HPV-31 and HPV-33 which are phytogenetically related to HPV-16, and HPV-45 which is related to HPV-18. Analysis of a phase-3 clinical trial at four year-follow up showed that the vaccine efficacy against CIN3 regardless of HPV types among HPV-naïve girls/young women below 25-years old was 93.4%, and among all participants regardless of history of HPV exposure, was 65%. The serum antibody levels for both HPV-16 and HPV-18 are sustained for more than 10 years to confer long-term protection of vaccinated women against these HPV infections.

Cervarix® is administered by intramuscular injection at month-0, month-1 and month-6 except in adolescent girls below 15-years old, who need only two doses. The second dose at month-1 is omitted.

(ii) Gardasil®

This is a HPV6/11/16/18 quadrivalent vaccine using aluminum hydroxide as the adjuvant compound. HPV-6 and HPV-11 are non-oncogenic but are responsible for almost 90% of genital warts. The immunogenicity of the vaccine is good but cross protection against other oncogenic HPV is low. In phase-3 clinical trials, the vaccine efficacy against CIN3 regardless of HPV types among HPV-naïve girls/young women below 26-years old was 43%, and among all participants regardless of history of HPV exposure, was 19%.

Gardasil® is administered in a similar manner as Cervarix® except the second dose is given at month-2. A two-dose regimen is also recommended for adolescent girls below 14-years old, by omitting the month-2 dose.

(iii) Gardasil-9

This is a second generation HPV vaccine from the same manufacturer as for Gardasil®. Compared to Gardasil®, this newly available HPV vaccine has protection of additional five high-risk HPV subtypes. It covers HPV6/11/16/18/31/35/45/52/58. The range of HPV protection covers HPV subtypes that are found in 90% of cervical cancers. Studies on the immunogenicity of the vaccine have demonstrated excellent serum antibody levels against vaccine targeted HPV subtypes with 100% vaccine efficacy against CIN3 from vaccine-targeted HPV subtypes. There is no information on the efficacy against CIN3 regardless of HPV types. Also, there is no comparison study between Gardasil-9 and Cervarix® on protection rate against CIN3 regardless of HPV types.

The administration of Gardasil-9 follows the schedule recommended for Gardasil®.

Selected Diseases

1. Cervical Cancer

Globally, cervical cancer ranks the fourth among the most common cancers in women with more than 600,000 new cases diagnosed each year. Approximately one half of cervical cancer patients die from the disease. The incidence rate and mortality rate of cervical cancer vary according to the economic status of the country. Almost 80% of the global burden and mortality of cervical cancer occurs in developing countries because of lack of resources for screening and treatment. In Singapore, both the incidence and mortality rates of cervical cancer have declined in the last four decades. It ranks the 10th among the most common cancers in women and the 8th in the cause of mortality in women. The mean age of women diagnosed with cervical cancer is 45-years.

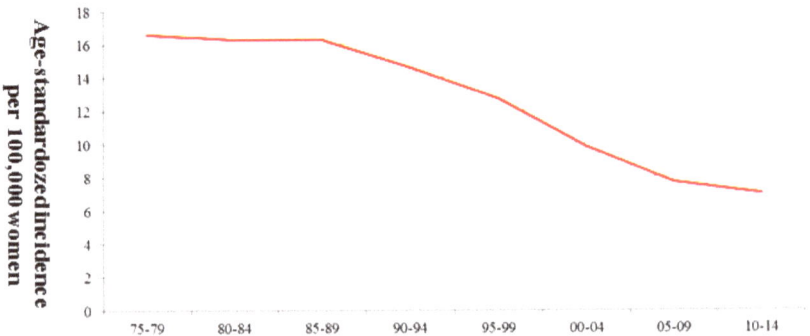

This chart shows the trend of incidence of cervical cancer in Singapore from 1975 to 2014.

Human papillomavirus (HPV) subtypes 16, 18, 31, 33, 35, 39, 45, 51, 52, 56, 58, 59, 68 are the high-risk or oncogenic HPV. There are responsible for 95–99% of all cervical cancer. High-risk HPV, via E6 and E7 viral oncoproteins, plays an essential part in neoplastic transformation in the cervix. The intracellular p53 and retinoblastoma (Rb) proteins are depleted by increased degradation of p53-E6 and Rb-E7 complexes. The neoplastic transformation occurs with persistent virus infection. In the great majority of cases, HPV infection is a transient phenomenon with no neoplastic consequences.

The other independent risk factors for cervical cancer include initiation of sexual intercourse during the teen age, multiparity, chronic immunosuppression or immunodeficiency, and tobacco smoking.

Primary cervical cancers are predominantly (75%) squamous cell carcinoma and adenocarcinoma (20%), and less commonly adenosquamous cell carcinoma (<5%). These are HPV-related cancers. Rare tumors of the cervix which are not related to HPV infection include the intestinal variant of adenocarcinoma, melanoma, adenosarcoma, rhabdomyosarcoma, and lymphoma. Uterine cervix is an uncommon site for secondary or metastatic cancer except direct spread of endometrial carcinoma and, less commonly, metastatic breast cancer.

Cervical cancer is a slowly growing tumor with local extension of the tumor along the parametrial tissues and uterosacral ligaments which share the same embryological compartment as the cervix. The tumor can also extend into the vagina to reach and go beyond the introitus. It invades the bladder anteriorly and rectum posteriorly, forming vesicovaginal and/or rectovaginal fistulae. It permeates and is disseminated in lymphatic system along the pelvic vessels and nerves in the early phase of the disease. It is also disseminated through the hematogenous route to distant sites such as the lungs, liver and bone.

Signs and symptoms of cervical cancer are absent in the early stages. They are detected on screening test. In the later stage of the disease, there may be increased vaginal discharge, post-coital bleeding, intermenstrual bleeding, or postmenopausal bleeding.

In locally advanced cases, there may be urinary leakage or vaginal fecal discharge from fistulae. Disseminated cases may present symptoms of the involved sites such as cough, bone pain, backache and lower limb edema. Occasionally, patients may present to other disciplines for chronic renal failure or urinary or fecal incontinence.

Cervical cancer is staged by the FIGO system into stages 1–4, according to clinical examination which include a bimanual examination of the cervix, uterus and pelvis, proto-sigmoidoscopy, cystoscopy, intravenous urography, and a chest X-ray.

- Stage-1A: No clinically visible tumor on the cervix. The invasive disease is based on histological examination and the dimension of the invasion is not more than 5 mm in depth and not more than 7 mm in breadth.
- Stage-1B: Microscopic cancer greater than stage-1A in dimensions or clinically visible tumor confined to the cervix.
- Stage-2A: Clinical tumor extending from the cervix to the upper one-half of the vagina.
- Stage-2B: Clinical tumor extending to parametrium but not reaching the pelvic side walls.
- Stage-3A: Tumor extending to the lower one-half of the vagina.
- Stage-3B: Tumor infiltrating the parametrium up to the pelvic side walls, or demonstration of hydroureter and/or hydronephrosis on radiology.
- Stage-4A: Tumor extending to the mucosal aspect of the bladder or rectum.
- Stage-4B: Tumor with extension or metastasis beyond the above description.

In advanced medical care centers, investigation with magnetic resonance imaging of the pelvis provides an excellent assessment of the extent of tumor loco-regionally, including tumor involvement in the lymphatic and urinary tracts. Computerized tomography (CT) scan of the thorax and abdomen also provides a good assessment of distant metastasis of the cancer. Alternatively, assessment of distant dissemination of the cancer can be done with a

FDG PET-CT body scan. This is a concomitant CT scan with a positron emission tomography (PET) with 2-deoxy-2-[fluorine-18] fluoro-D-glucose (^{18}F-FDG). ^{18}F-FDG scan detects cancerous cells which demonstrate an increased glucose uptake and glycolysis.

Other investigations relevant to cervical cancer care are full blood count for the management of anemia and renal panel for the management of renal function deficiency from obstructive uropathy.

Definitive treatment of cervical cancer depends on the stage of the cancer:

(i) Stage-1A: These cases tend to be found in young women who are keen to conserve the reproductive capability. The disease can be treated with conization of the cervix. In patients who have completed the family size or who have decided against childbearing, the disease is treated with a simple hysterectomy with conservation of the ovaries.

The alternative treatment for patients not fit for surgery or who have decided against surgery is radiotherapy.

(ii) Stage-1B and 2A: The standard surgical management is a radical hysterectomy with excision of the parametrial and uterosacral ligaments, and pelvic lymphadenectomy. In young women desirous of childbearing, the cancer can be treated with radical trachelectomy and pelvic lymphadenectomy. Radical trachelectomy involves amputation of the cervix at the level of the internal os and excision of the parametrial and uteroscaral ligaments as in radical hysterectomy.

The alternative treatment for patients not fit for surgery or who decide against surgery is concurrent chemoradiation, which confers an equal outcome as surgery.

(iii) Stage-2B and beyond: Surgical management is inadequate. Definitive treatment is by concurrent chemoradiation.

Prognosis of cervical cancer is good for the early stages. The five-year survival rate is 100% for stage-1A, 85% for stage-1B, 70% for stage-2A, 60% for stage-2B, 50% for stage-3A/B, 30% for stage-4A, and 10% for stage-4B.

The most common cause of death in cervical cancer is renal failure.

2. Cervical Intraepithelial Neoplasia (CIN)

Cervical carcinoma of the cervix is preceded by a pre-malignant phase by a decade. The pre-malignant lesions are neoplastic cells confined to the intraepithelial compartment of the epithelium, without breeching of the basement membrane. These cells manifest features of neoplasia: increased nuclear-cytoplasmic ratio, nuclear enlargement and hyperchromasia, increased abnormal mitosis, and reduced cytoplasmic maturation. The maturation process of epithelial cells from the basalis layer towards the superficialis layer of the epithelium is incomplete or totally loss as in the case of carcinoma *in situ*. The term cervical intraepithelial neoplasia or CIN has been in use since 1974.

Based on the proportion of epithelial thickness involved, CIN is classified in increasing severity into CIN grade-1 or CIN1, grade-2 or CIN2, and grade-3 or CIN3. CIN1 refers to the extent of neoplastic abnormalities confined to the basal one-third of the epithelium. CIN2 refers to the abnormal changes extending beyond one-third but less than two-thirds of the basal portion of the epithelium. CIN3 is diagnosed when the neoplasia involves more than two-thirds of the epithelial thickness. This definition of CIN3 encompasses the old terminology of carcinoma *in situ* which refers to neoplasia involving the full thickness of the epithelium.

CIN shares the same epidemiological features and HPV etiology as the invasive squamous cell carcinoma of the cervix, except HPV subtypes found in CIN is more heterogeneous than in squamous cell carcinoma. Low-risk HPV, such as HPV-6, can readily induce cytopathic changes of CIN1 and, less commonly, CIN2.

The natural history of CIN is well characterized. CIN1 is indistinguishable from cytopathic effects of HPV infection and carries a low potential of malignant progression. More than 70% of cases of

CIN1, in young women (<35 years old) in particular, regresses spontaneously. Spontaneous regression occurs in 50% of CIN2 and less than 25% of CIN3. On the other hand, the cumulative risk of progression of CIN3 to invasive carcinoma exceeds 50% over 25-years.

CIN does not present with any specific signs and symptoms. The cervix is generally normal in appearance to the naked eye and normal in consistency on digital palpation. Suspicion of the existence of CIN is raised by abnormal screening test.

In addition to neoplastic cellular changes and reduced glycogen content within the cytoplasm, CIN manifest tissue architectural changes microscopically, in particular, the increased neovasculature. These properties allow the neoplastic epithelium to be identified on examination under magnification, or colposcopy.

Colposcopy is a transvaginal examination of the cervix with a binocular operating microscope at magnification power of 3.75×, 7.5× and 15× and with a strong electric illumination. Once the cervix is washed with 5% acetic acid, the neoplastic epithelium displays the following characteristics:

- Acetowhite: a phenomenon of transient opacification of the epithelium.
- Mosaicism: the cobblestone appearance of the epithelium resembling mosaic pattern on a wall or on the floor. This is the effect of horizontally running capillaries on an opaque background.
- Punctation: this is an appearance of small red dots scattered on the opaque epithelium. The red dots are the end-on appearance of vertically running capillary loops.
- Atypical blood vessels: a haphazard display of irregular neovasculature.

CIN manifests its increasing severity with increasing density of opacity, coarseness of mosaic pattern and punctuation, and presence of atypical blood vessels.

Loss of cellular glycogen content allows CIN in estrogenized (premenopausal) epithelium to be identified as loss of dark brown staining areas after application of iodine on the cervix.

The objectives of colposcopy are:

- Confirmation and localization of CIN on the cervix
- Assessment of CIN severity by the characteristic features on colposcopy
- Directed biopsies from the most severe areas for histological diagnosis
- Adjunct to treatment procedure for CIN.

Curative treatment of CIN is by surgical eradication of the affected transformation zone of the cervix. Several modalities are effective and the common procedures are:

- *Loop electro-excision procedure (LEEP).* A metal wire loop mounted on a hand piece is heated with a surgical electro-diathermy device and is used to excise the target tissue. Loops of varying diameters are available to suit the dimension of tissue excision desired. This is an office procedure done with intracervical injection of a local anesthetic agent. The excised tissue is subjected to histopathologic assessment for definitive diagnosis and completeness of the excision of CIN.

- *Cervical conization or cone biopsy.* In this procedure, complete excision of the transformation zone begins with a broad base at the ectocervix and the excision proceeds circumferentially and converged towards the internal os. The excised tissue assumes a conical shape. This procedure can be done with a cold knife under regional or general anesthesia, or CO_2 laser which can be done with a paracervical local anesthetic. Conization is generally done for CIN3 with extension of the disease into the endocervical canal or for cases where colposcopy suspects an early invasive carcinoma. Definitive histopathologic diagnosis and completeness of the excision of the lesion can be assured.

- *CO_2 laser vaporization of transformation zone.* This is an office procedure performed under paracervical anesthetic. No tissue is available for histology confirmation of CIN and its completeness of eradication.

- *Cryotherapy.* Liquid nitrogen is applied onto the transformation zone of the cervix via an applicator. The freeze-thaw process causes destruction of the targeted tissue. This is a low cost office procedure done without the need for anesthesia. No surgical tissue is available for confirmation of histological diagnosis or completeness of CIN eradication.

3. Adenocarcinoma *In situ* (AIS)

This is an *in situ* carcinoma arising from the endocervical glandular epithelium. It is a HPV-related condition and co-exists with CIN in 50% of cases. It is a precursor lesion of adenocarcinoma of the cervix. Unlike CIN, which is mostly a surface lesion, AIS involves glands which extends deep into the cervical stromal tissue, and for some cases, extends close to the lower part of the endometrial cavity.

AIS does not present with any specific signs and symptoms. It is suspected on screening or diagnosed incidentally on excisional treatment of CIN.

Treatment of AIS is by conization of the cervix for women desirous of fertility or by hysterectomy. Local ablative treatment with CO_2 laser vaporization or cryotherapy is inappropriate as the completeness of eradication of the lesion cannot be assured. In women who do not desire to conserve reproductive capability, a simple total hysterectomy is the standard of care for AIS.

Illustrations of Cervical Cancer and Pre-malignant Diseases

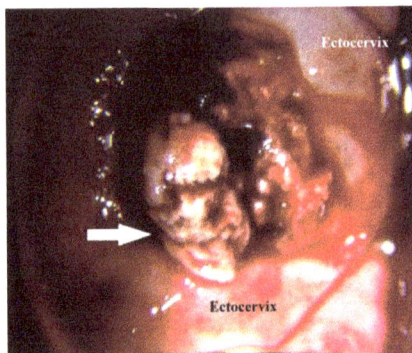

This photograph shows a friable tumor (pointed out by the white arrow) at the external os of the cervix.

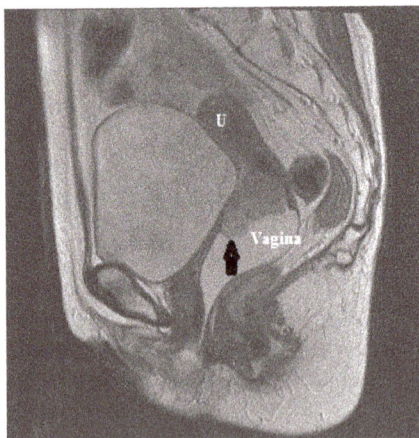

This photograph of a sagittal section of MR image shows a cervical tumor extending to the upper portion of the anterior vagina wall (black arrow). The vagina was filled with gel for anatomical illustration of the anatomy. The uterus is identified by "U". This 45-year-old was diagnosed with a stage-IIA carcinoma of the cervix.

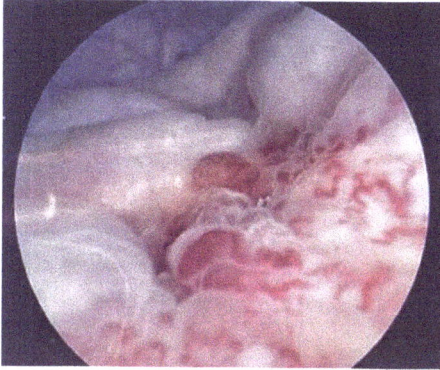

This woman had a cystoscopy as part of surgical staging of the carcinoma of the cervix. Tumor invasion of the bladder mucosa as shown in this photograph was confirmed on histology of the biopsies.

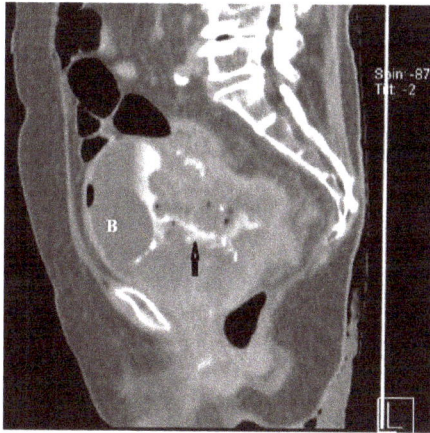

This photograph of a section of post-contrast CT-scan shows a fistula tract (black arrow) between bladder (marked "B") and the uterus, in a woman with a locally advanced carcinoma of the cervix.

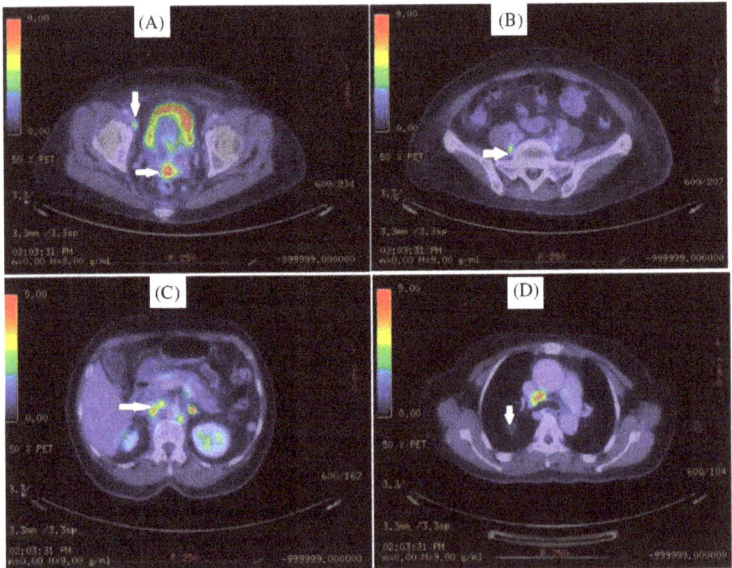

This woman was investigated with a PET-CT scan for a primary cervical cancer. The photographs shows FDG avid uptake at the primary tumor on the cervix (panel A), common iliac lymph node (panel B), aorto-caval lymph node (panel C) and lung (panel D).

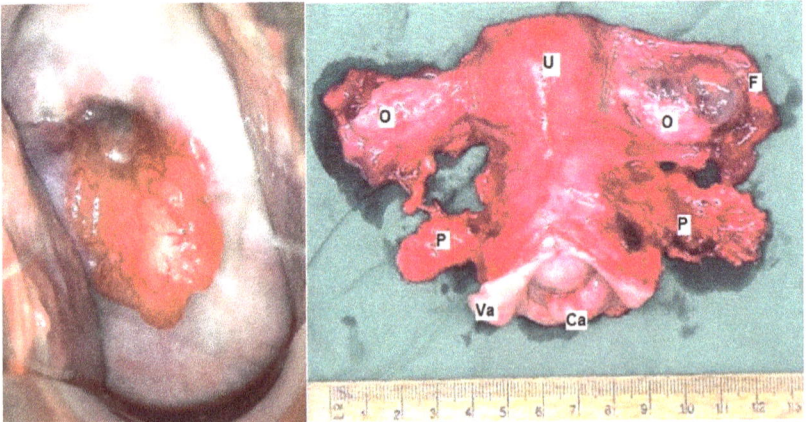

This 50-year-old woman had a stage-IB cervical cancer (panel left) and undertook a radical hysterectomy (panel right). U = Uterus; O = ovaries; Ca = Cervical tumor; Va = vagina; P = parametrium.

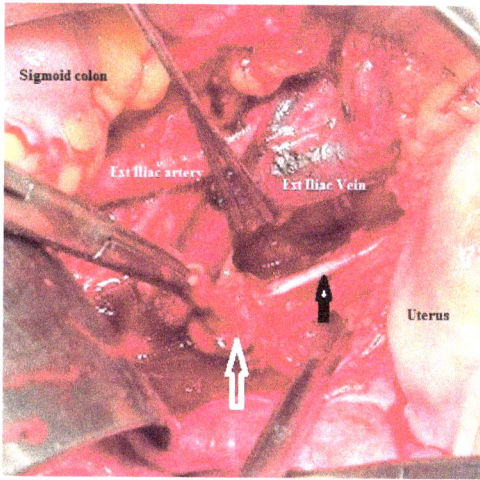

This photograph shows the retroperitoreal structures revealed during pelvic lymphadenectomy for radical hysterectomy for cervical cancer. The black arrow points to the obturator nerve and the white arrow points to fat pad of obturator lymph nodes.

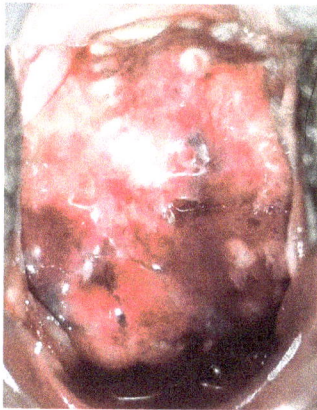

This 42-year-old woman complained of profuse watery vaginal discharge for 3 months. She had multiple negative cytology screening tests in the preceding 12 years. The last screening was 10 months previous to the present complaint. On examination, a large exophytic tumor was seen to have replaced the entire cervix. The tumor was irregular and had a few small pigmented areas. This was a case of primary melanoma of the cervix, an extremely rare primary tumor of the cervix.

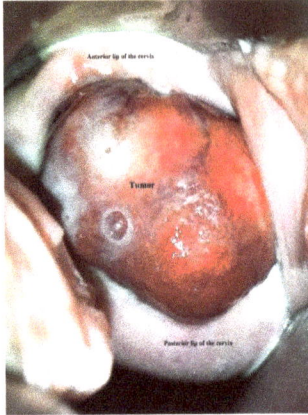

This 40-year-old woman complained of prolonged vaginal bleeding. Her cervical screening 12 months previously was negative for intraepithelial neoplasia and malignancy. She was noted to have a large tumor distending the cervical os. The anterior and posterior lips of the cervix were seen as a firm rim of tissue embracing the tumor. This tumor was confirmed to be a leiomyoma on excision biopsy.

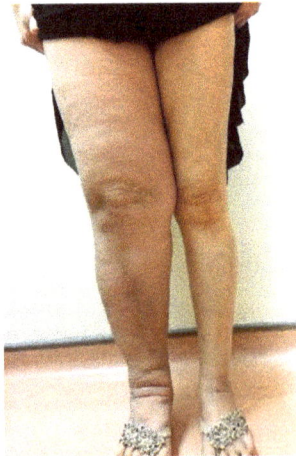

This photograph shows a woman with chronic lymphedema of the right lower limb following radical hysterectomy and bilateral pelvic lymphadenectomy 10 years previously.

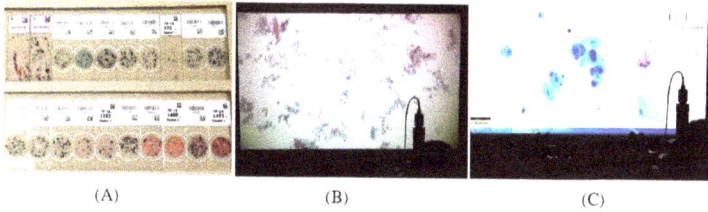

(A)   (B)   (C)

This photographs shows cytology laboratory screening: panel (A) shows a tray of monolayer preparations of liquid-based cytology; panels (B) and (C) show low and high power fields on microscopy of the cells.

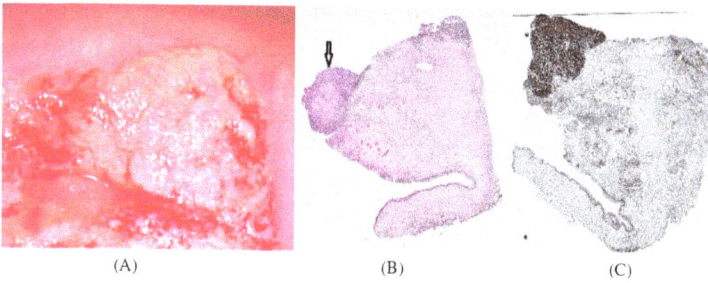

(A)   (B)   (C)

This 43-year-old woman had a cervical screening showing HSIL. On colposcopy, there was a raised and irregular lesion on the cervix (panel A). Histology confirmed the tumor on routine hematoxylin and Eosin staining (panel B) and p16 immunohistochemical staining (panel C).

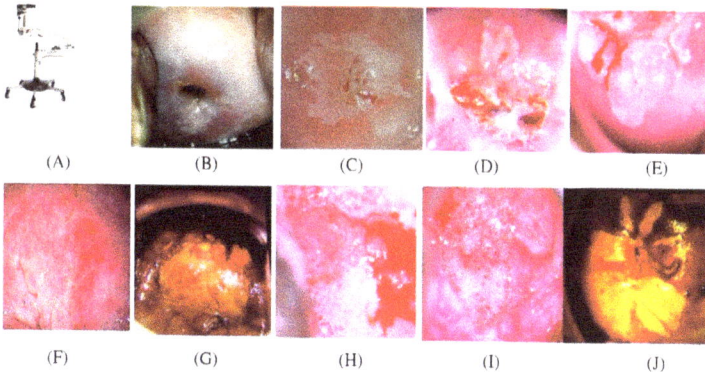

(A)   (B)   (C)   (D)   (E)

(F)   (G)   (H)   (I)   (J)

These colpophotos show the features of CIN: acetowhite, mosaicism, punctuation and atypical blood vessels. (A): binocular colposcope; (B&C): Cervical HPV infection; (D): CIN1; (E): CIN2; (F & G): CIN3; (H & I): Microinvasive cancer; (J): Iodine staining showing HPV infection.

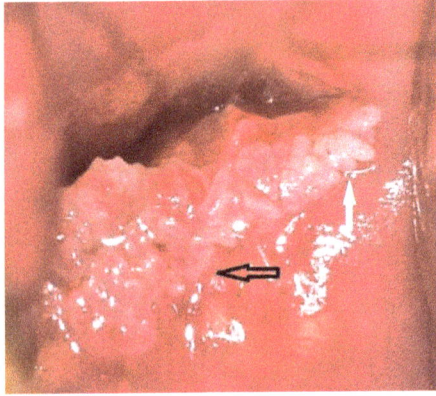

This young woman with LSIL was found on colposcopy to have a cervical condyloma (black open arrow) and a small area of acetowhite (white solid arrow) consistent of CIN1. HPV type 6 is the most common cause of condyloma acuminate. It can also cause CIN1 and some CIN2.

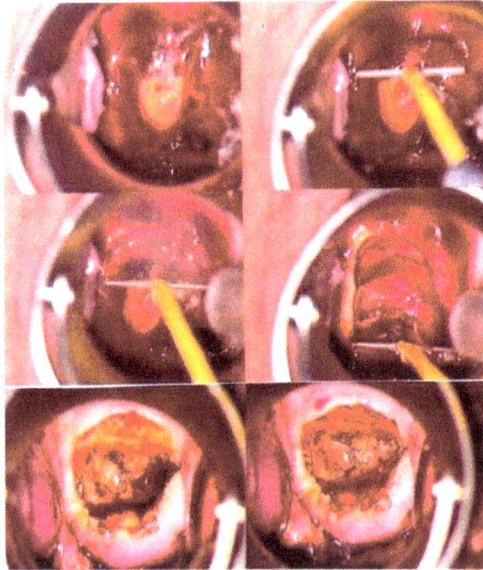

This panel of photographs shows the treatment of CIN using loop-electro-excision procedure (LEEP). The entire transformation zone of the cervix was excised. The device combines the function of cutting and coagulation to reduce the bleeding during the procedure.

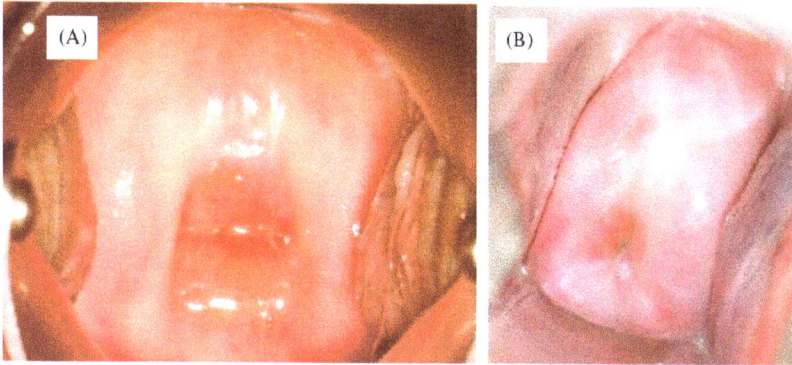

This panel of photographs shows the effect on the cervix after LEEP. In panel (A), the cervix healed with a patulous external os. In panel (B), the cervix of this post-menopausal woman had become stenotic.

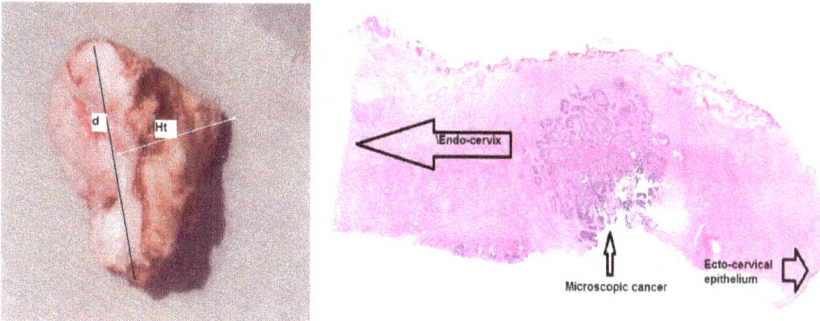

This 45-year-old woman was tested positive for HPV-16, but the cytology was negative. A colposcopy showed a lesion in the endocervix but was deemed technically unsatisfactory as the lesion could not be seen in entirety. She undertook a cone biopsy (panel on the left: the length of cone biopsy — Ht and the width — d were tailored according to the suspected location and size of the lesion). In this case, pathology examination found a small invasive cancer on the endocervix (panel on the right).

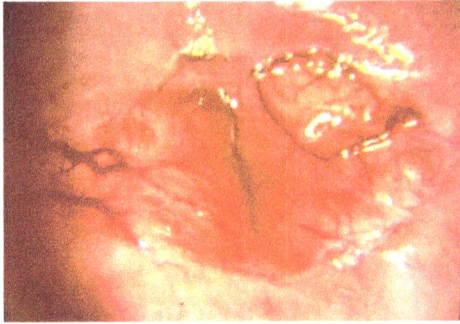

This elderly woman was investigated for vaginal discharge. The LBC was negative for intraepithelial neoplasia and malignancy. She was found to have prominent vessels on the cervix. This feature is normal for a cervix showing severe epithelial thinning from menopausal atrophy.

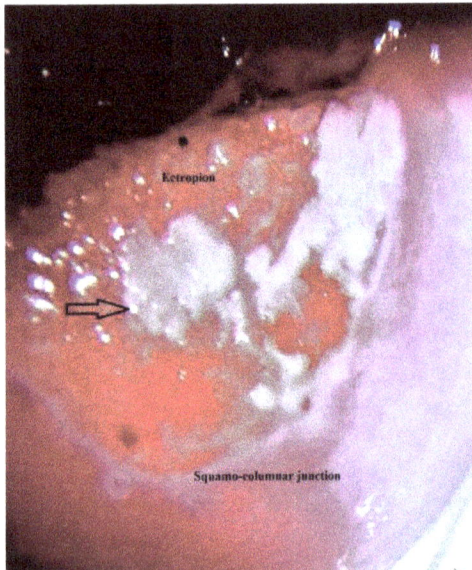

This 48-year-old was asymptomatic. Her LBC showed adenocarcinoma *in situ*. On colposcopy, a slightly raised and intensely acetowhite lesion was seen within the ectropion area of the cervix (open arrow). This lesion was confirmed.

CASE 21 — SUBFERTILITY

A 32-year-old woman has not conceived after trying for 12 months.

- When does failure to conceive become a clinical problem?
- What are the common causes of subfertility in women?
- What are the male factors in failure to conceive?
- What assisted reproductive techniques are currently available?

When does Failure to Conceive Become a Clinical Problem?

Pregnancy is a personal objective. Some couples wish to achieve a pregnancy as soon as they attempt it, while others would let nature take its cause. They may seek medical professional opinion and management according to their individual objectives.

Physiologically, the probability of a woman conceiving following sexual intercourse during peri-ovulatory phase is 20% per cycle, with a cumulative pregnancy rate of 66% at six months and 85% at 12 months. Pregnancy rate decreases with increasing duration of not conceiving. Customarily, failure to conceive after 12 months of active attempts is considered a clinical problem that warrants investigations to identify the underlying explanations. The duration of 12 months is arbitrary and early investigation is warranted in older women who, because of the natural decline in age-related fertility rate, are more likely to require artificial reproductive assistance.

What are the Common Causes of Subfertility in Women?

The female reproductive physiology for pregnancy involves (1) ovulation; (2) transporting of the ovum to the ampulla portion of the fallopian tube for fertilization; (3) transporting of fertilized gamete to the uterine cavity; and (4) endometrial implantation of the embryo.

Female factor alone contributes to 35% and combined female and male factor contributes to 20% of subfertility cases. The known female factors, which may be single or multiple in one individual case, include:

(i) **Cervical factors**
   - Stenosis: scarring from previous surgery, infection, or radiation
   - Abnormal mucus-sperm interaction: qualitative and quantitative dysfunction of cervical mucus

(ii) **Uterine factors**
   - Congenital anomaly: Mayer-Rokitansky-Küster-Hauser (MRKH) syndrome
   - Asherman syndrome
   - Fibroids: submucous or intrauterine
   - Adenomyosis

(iii) **Ovarian factors: anovulation**
   - Polycystic ovarian syndrome
   - Hyperprolactinemia
   - Thyroid dysfunctions
   - Pre-mature ovarian failure
   - Sex chromosomal aberrations
   - Weight change-related hypothalamic-pituitary axis dysfunction

(iv) **Tubal factors**
   - Blocked fallopian tubes: hydrosalpinx, salpingitis, tubal ligation, post-surgery
   - Salpingectomy

(v)   **Peritoneal factors**
  • Adhesions (post-surgical, infection, endometriosis)
(vi) **Advanced age**
  • Infertility rate starts to rise after the age of 35-years of age, reaching 33% after 40-years and 87% after 45-years.

What are the Male Factors in Failure to Conceive?

Male factor alone contributes to 35% of subfertility cases. The most commonly (90%) encountered problems are low sperm counts, and poor sperm quality or both. The male reproductive process involves formation and transportation of sperms. Abnormality in sperm formation can be pre-testicular or testicular in origin while sperm transportation problem is post-testicular in origin.

(i)   **Pre-testicular factors** or hypothalamic-pituitary axis aberration
  • Hyperprolactinemia
  • Hypogonadotropic hypogonadism (Idiopathic, *Laurence-Moon-Biedl syndrome, Prader-Willi syndrome*)
  • CNS tumors, temporal lobe seizures
  • Isolated LH insufficiency
  • Isolated FSH insufficiency

(ii) **Testicular factors**: primary testicular failure may result from chromosomal or non-chromosomal abnormalities

  Chromosomal
  • Y-chromosome microdeletions (azoospermia or severe oligozoospermia)
  • Klinefelter Syndrome : 47XXY (azoospermia)
  • XYY male
  • *Noonan syndrome (46, XY)*
  • *Mixed gonadal dysgenesis (45, X/46, XY)*

  Non-chromosomal
  • Idiopathic

- Gonadotoxic drugs
- Radiation
- Orchitis
- Trauma
- Torsion

(iii) Post-testicular factors

Congenital ductal abnormalities:

- Absence of vas deferens
- Duct obstruction from pre-natal maternal exposure to diethylstilbestrol (DES)
- Cystic fibrosis

Acquired ductal obstruction:

- Infections (chlamydia, gonorrhea, and tuberculosis)
- Surgery (vasectomy, hydrocelectomy and spermato-celectomy)
- *Ejaculatory duct obstruction* (cysts, ductal calcification and stones, post infectious, and postoperative)
- Anejaculation/retrograde ejaculation

What Assisted Reproductive Techniques are Currently Available?

The aim of treatment of subfertility is to expedite a couple's fulfilment of the objective to conceive. The exact treatments are based on the etiology of subfertility, but a significant number of couple would require the help of assisted reproductive technologies (ART). ART is a collective term for various technologies in which eggs and sperm are handled outside the body. The most well-established and widely used ART include the following:

• Intrauterine Insemination (IUI)

IUI involves the placement of sperm directly into the uterus. After laboratory processing, sperms, with an insemination motile count of 1 million or above, are injected into the uterine cavity via a transcervical cannula. The timing of insemination is immediately before and not more than 10 hours after ovulation. The pregnancy rate per cycle of insemination has been reported to be 4% if used alone and 8–17% if combined with superovulation. The cumulative pregnancy rates are similar for six cycles of IUI, three cycles of IVF with single embryo transfer, and six cycles of modified natural cycle IVF.

IUI is the treatment of choice for couples who have unexplained subfertility, cervical mucus hostility towards sperms, mild endometriosis, and male factors with reasonably good sperm quality, and in couples with sexual disorders such as vaginismus and erectile dysfunction.

• *In vitro* Fertilization (IVF)

After controlled ovarian hyperstimulation with injections of gonadotrophins, the oocytes are retrieved from the ovaries and incubated in laboratory condition for a period of three to six hours. Approximately 100,000 motile sperm per oocyte are then added to the medium for fertilization outside the body. After 48 hours, the embryos have usually reached the 3- to 8-cell stage and one or two embryos are transferred into the uterine cavity via a transcervical cannula. Pregnancy rates are 10–45%.

IVF is a safe and well-established assisted reproductive procedure since 1978. It is associated with a 5% risk of ovarian hyperstimuation syndrome. The rate of multiple gestations is approximately 5%. There is a slightly higher risk of birth defects, most notably a 0.3–1.5% risk of hypospadias in male neonates.

• Intracytoplasmic Sperm Injection (ICSI)

In contrast to spontaneous fertilization *in vitro* (IVF), ICSI involves the direct injection of a sperm into an oocyte under microscopy. Sperms from ejaculation or from surgical retrieval from testicles are assessed for their motility, morphology, and DNA quality. The most appropriate sperm is picked up with a micropipette and carefully injected into the cytoplasm of an oocyte which has been processed with hyaluronidase to remove the cumulus mass and corona radiata. After incubation for 48 hours, the embryo transfer into the woman's uterus is carried out.

The fertilization and pregnancy rate is approximately 60% and 35%, respectively, regardless of fresh or cryopreserved sperms. It is indicated in patients with sperm deficiencies, including sperm extracted directly from the epididymis or testicle. It is also indicated for patients who have not conceived with other methods of treatment.

Selected Disease

Pelvic Inflammatory Diseases

Pelvic inflammatory disease (PID) refers to infection of the upper genital tract, namely endometritis, salpingitis, oophoritis and pelvic peritonitis. The exact incidence of PID is unknown but, in the USA, they accounted for approximately 150,000 hospital admissions each year.

With a few exceptions of hematogenous spread of bacteria and infection following pelvic surgery, such as insertion of intrauterine device (IUD), dilatation and curettage, laparoscopy and laparotomy, the great majority of PID results from ascending infection from the vagina and, generally, are related to sexual transmissions.

The most common primary cause of PID is sexually transmitted infection (STI) by either chlamydia trachomatis or Neisseria gonorrhea. These infections may be followed by concomitant polymicrobial infections with Gardnerella vaginalis, Haemophilus influenzae, Ureaplasma, and anaerobes such as Peptococcus and Bacteroides species.

The risk factors of STI-related PID are:

- Young age, particularly below 25-years old
- First sexual intercourse

- Multiple sexual partners
- Lives in area with high prevalence of STI
- Do not use contraception

PID is associated with three significant complications:

(i) Chronic pelvic pain: this complication is estimated to occur in 25% of acute PID.
(ii) Infertility: salpingitis causes scarring and adhesions within tubal lumens and results in infertility from tubal factor in 15% of cases after one episode of PID. The rate of infertility increases with the number of episodes of infection.
(iii) Ectopic pregnancy: women with a history of PID face a 15–50% risk of ectopic pregnancy.

Signs and symptoms

- Both chlamydia and gonorrhea infection may be asymptomatic, though gonorrhea is more often symptomatic compared to chlamydia infection
- Most cases of PID have an onset towards the end of menstruation or within the first 10 days of menstruation
- Gonococcal PID may present abruptly with toxic symptoms of fever ≥38°C, nausea, vomiting, and severe pelvic and abdominal pain
- Non-gonococcal PID may present with a dull or aching constant lower abdominal pain
- Abnormal vaginal discharge, particularly mucopurulent discharge, is present in 75% of cases
- Post-coital bleeding is present in 40% of cases
- Abdominal tenderness with or without rebound tenderness
- Right upper quadrant tenderness: Fitz-Hugh–Curtis syndrome occurs in 4% of those with mild-to-moderate PID
- Cervical motion tenderness
- Uterine tenderness
- Adnexal tenderness.

Diagnosis and laboratory investigations

Diagnosis of PID is based on clinical presentation of the condition. There is no one single test that is diagnostic of PID. However, supportive diagnostic tests include:

- Hematological indices: leukocytosis occurs in <50% of acute PID. ESR is more sensitive than white cell counts
- Gonorrhea DNA probes and cultures
- Chlamydial vulvovaginal or endocervical DNA probes and cultures
- Transvaginal ultrasound scan:

    Positive findings on ultrasound scan in PID may include the following:
    — Echo thickening and heterogeneity in the central-endometrial-cavity suggestive of endometritis
    — Detection of hydrosalpinx
    — Enlarged ovaries with ill-defined margins and detection of free fluid in the adnexa or cul-de-sac
    — Detection of tubo-ovarian abscess: complex adnexal masses with thickened walls and central fluid

- Laparoscopic confirmation in cases not responding to antibiotic treatment.

Management of PID

Treatment of PID aims to relief acute symptoms, eradicate current infection, and minimize the risk of long-term sequelae. Early intervention is critical for preservation of fertility.

All uncomplicated PID cases are managed in the out-patient setting with broad-spectrum antibiotics to cover the full complement of common organisms and, in particular, *C. trachomatis* and *N. gonorrhoeae*. The recommended choice of antibiotic regimen consists of the following combination:

(i) Ceftriaxone 250 mg intramuscularly (IM) once as a single dose, or Cefoxitin 2 g IM once as a single dose concurrently with probenecid 1 g orally in a single dose, or another single-dose parenteral third-generation cephalosporin (e.g. cefti-zoxime or cefotaxime)

(ii) Doxycycline 100 mg orally twice daily for 14 days

(iii) Metronidazole 500 mg orally twice daily for 14 days for patients with suspected vaginitis or who had undertaken gynecologic instrumentation in the preceding two to three weeks

Almost 75% of PID, including 60% of tubo-ovarian abscesses, resolved with antibiotic treatment. Unresolved abscesses may be managed by computed tomographic (CT) or ultrasonography guided drainage either percutaneously or via posterior colpotomy.

In-patient treatment is sometimes indicated for the following situations:

- Diagnosis is uncertain
- Presence of pelvic abscess
- Patient is ill
- Pregnancy
- Inability to tolerate outpatient oral antibiotic regimen
- Immunodeficiency
- Failure to improve clinically after 72 hours of outpatient therapy

Role of Laparoscopy

Laparoscopy is preferred to laparotomy. It is indicated for patients whose diagnosis is in doubt or whose symptoms do not improve after 72 hours of out-patient treatment. In addition to diagnostic purpose, the surgery aims to conserve reproductive potential. The procedure should be limited to simple drainage, adhesiolysis, copious irrigation of the pelvis and, rarely, unilateral adnexectomy.

Illustration of Some Conditions Related to Subfertility

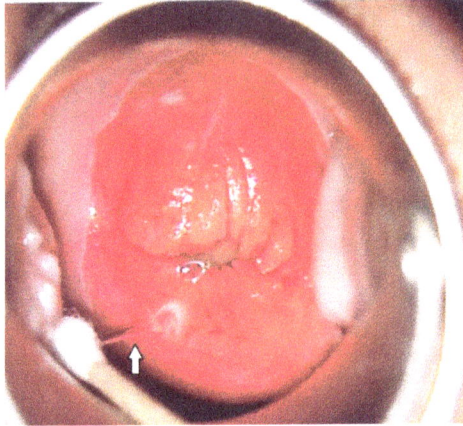

Anovulation is a common cause of subfertility. This photograph shows the cervix with a large ectropion in a young woman. The clear stretchy cervical mucus (white arrow) was indicative of the periovulatory timing of her menstrual cycle. Measurement of the length of the stretched mucus was used as a test for ovulation in the era when serum progesterone assay was not readily available.

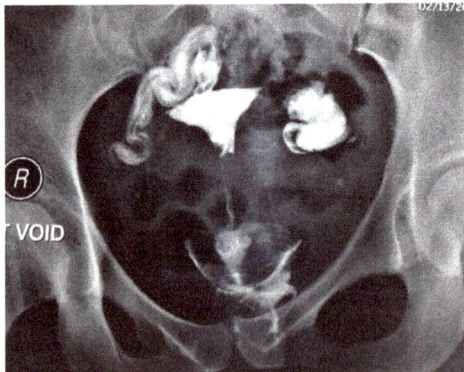

This photograph of a hysterosalpingogram (HSG) shows tubal blockade as the cause of infertility.

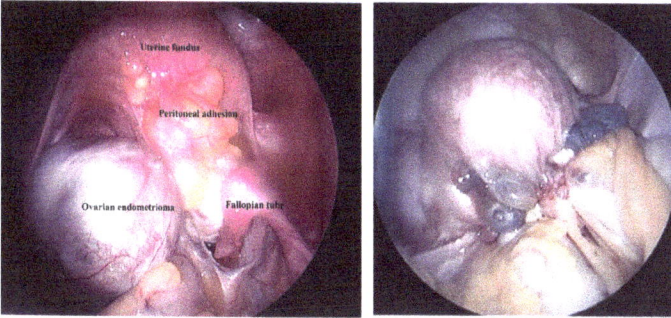

These photographs of a laparoscopy reveal severe pelvic endometriosis which is a common cause of subfertility.

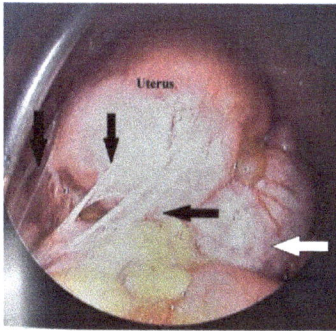

This photograph of a laparoscopy shows a case of PID with hydrosalpinx (white arrow) and dense and flimsy adhesions (black arrows) which obliterated the Pouch of Uterus.

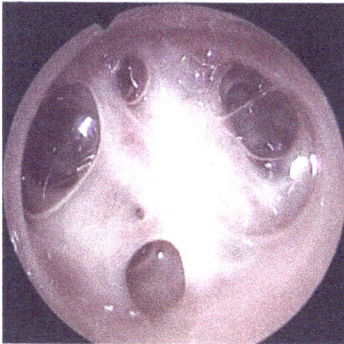

This photograph of a hysteroscopy shows severe fibrotic scarring in the uterine cavity (Asherman syndrome) which was the uterine factor for infertility in this woman.

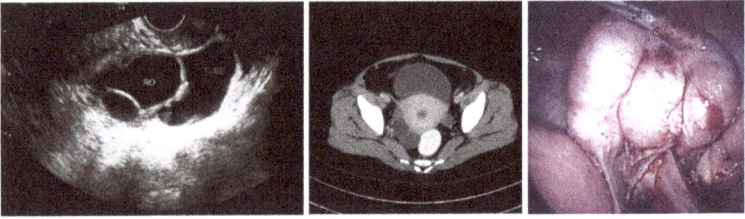

This panel of images shows hydrosalpinx as dilated tubal structure on ultrasound scan (left), CT-scan (middle panel) and on laparoscopy.

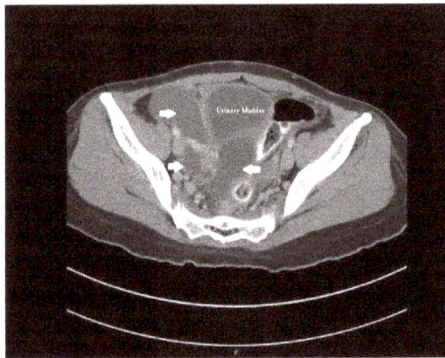

This photograph of a section of CT-scan demonstrates abscess collection in the pelvis (marked by white arrows).

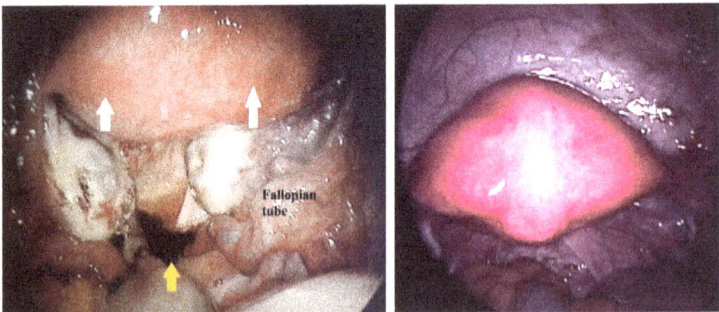

These photographs of laparoscopy show: on the left, a bicornuated uterus (marked by white arrows). Hydrotubation showed patent fallopian tubes with spillage of methylene blue solution from the fimbrial ends of the tubes (marked by yellow arrow). The uterus on the right showed the typical external appearance of a bicornuated uterus with a fibrotic band on the midline of the uterus. Bicornuated uterus is compatible for pregnancy.

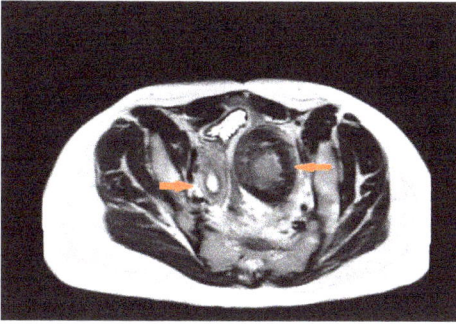

This photograph of a section of MR imaging study (T2 signal) shows the two horns (marked by the yellow arrows) of a bicornuated uterus.

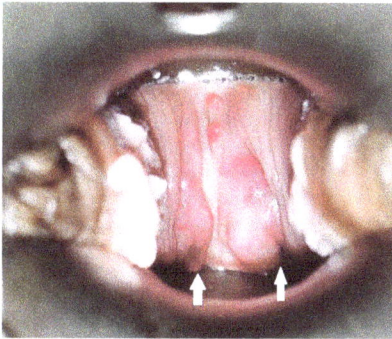

This photograph shows a congenital anomaly of the genital tract. There two cervices (marked by white arrows).

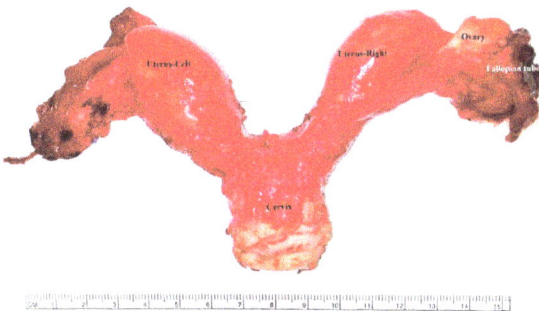

This photograph shows a hysterectomy specimen from Uteri Didelphys.

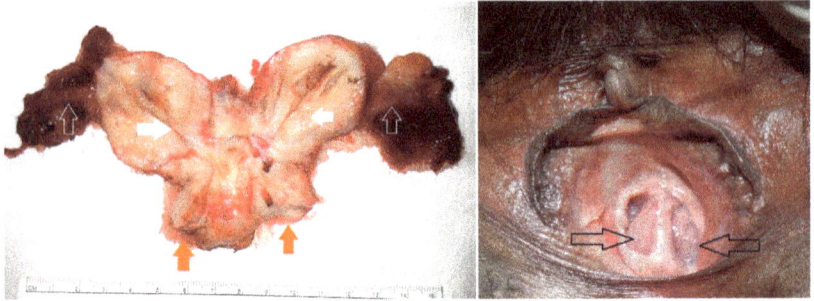

This panel of photographs shows an open specimen of a double uterus, also known as uteri didelfys, a congenital anomaly of the uterus where the two müllerian tubes failed to coalesce during the embryonic development. There were two uterine bodies (marked by white solid arrows) with a fallopian tube attached to each side (marked by open arrows), and two cervices (marked by yellow arrows). The panel on the right shows that there was also a double vagina (marked by open black arrows). Fully developed uteri didelfys is compatible with normal pregnancy as it happened in this case. Some cases of uteri didelfys are associated with recurrent miscarriages, premature deliveries or breech presentation of the fetus.

CASE 22 — FERTILITY CONTROL

A 30-year-old woman wants to delay a pregnancy.

- What reliable methods of contraception are available for her?
- What is post-coital contraception?
- What options does she have when an unplanned pregnancy occurs?

General Note

Contraception is an active and voluntary choice of the patient. In an accommodating and non-judgemental environment, the patient is counseled on the use, benefits and risks, and follow-up regimen of all methods of contraception. Experience and methods of previous contraception should be taken into consideration in assisting the patient to choose a method of contraception. Limited physical examination with blood pressure and weight monitoring, and a pelvic examination before IUD, is necessary. If reasonably certain of no pregnancy, the woman can start her choice of contraception immediately. Contraception should continue until menopause or until the woman reaches at least 50–55 years old.

What Reliable Methods of Contraception are Available for her?

Reliable methods of contraception are available to suit individual patient's objective: short-term reversible, long-term reversible and permanent contraception.

(i) Oral Contraceptive Pills (OCP)

OCP is taken in a 28-day cycle consisting of single daily dose for 21 days and a seven-day pill-free or placebo interval between the cycles. It is the most reliable short-term contraception with a reported contraceptive failure rate of 0.5 events/100 woman-year (95% CI: 0.4–0.5). The challenge of OCP lies in compliance of its use in terms of missed pills and continuation of pills in the subsequent cycles. There is also a possibility of interference in its gastrointestinal absorption by concurrent medications used for intercurrent illnesses. These challenges lead to a contraceptive failure rate of 9% in real world experience.

The reversibility of contraception is assured by findings that approximately 89% of women conceive within two years of cessation of OCP. The cumulative conception rate is not different from non-users after adjusting for age.

OCP has a good menstrual cycle control. OCP users, compared to non-users, are shown to have a lower risk of ovarian cyst formation, and lower life-time risk of ovarian and endometrial cancer.

The adverse effects of OCP are based on the biological activities of the component hormones. The most widely used OCP contains ethinylestradiol, either at 20 µg or 30 µg, and a progestin. All progestins are derivatives of 19-nortestosterone, except drospirenone which is a derivative of 17α-spironolactone. The table below shows the classification of progestins according to their generation of development.

Generation	Preparation	Progestational Activity	Estrogenic Activity	Androgenic Activity
First	Norethindrone	low	low	low
	Ethynodiol diacetate	moderate	low	low
Second	Levonorgestrel	high	low	high
	Norgestrel	high	high	high
Third	Desogestrel	high	low	low
	Norgestimate	high	low	low
Fourth	Drospirenone	high	low	low

The difference in the progestational, estrogenic and androgenic property between the molecules determines their pharmacological profile and side effects. The ideal OCP is one with high progestational activity and low in estrogenic and androgenic activities.

Minor gastrointestinal side effects are common, including nausea, vomiting, stomach cramps, bloating, diarrhea or constipation, increased or decreased appetite and weight gain or weight loss. There may be skin changes with brown or black patches, acne or hair growth in unusual places. Menstrual changes may occur with bleeding or spotting between menstrual periods, changes in menstrual flow, or painful or missed periods. They may be dizziness or faintness, breast tenderness and enlargement, and some experience an increase in white vaginal discharge.

Uncommon but more serious side effects of OCP that should prompt urgent medical attention includes severe headache, speech problems, weakness or numbness of an arm or leg, leg pain, partial or complete loss of vision, double vision, bulging eyes, crushing chest pain or chest heaviness, coughing up blood, shortness of breath, dark-colored urine and light-colored stool, or depression.

Mild and reversible increase in systolic and diastolic blood pressure is seen in some OCP users. The absolute risk of venous thrombo-embolism (VTE) is low, estimated to be between 1 in 100,000 and 1 in 300,000. The first three months of OCP use are the most at risk period because of the potential underlying hereditary and acquired risk of VTE. The other risk factors include advancing age, obesity and cigarette smoking. The modern OCP containing less than 50 μg of ethinylestradiol does not increase the risk of myocardial infarction among healthy users without other cardiovascular risk factors. The small additional risk of ischemic stroke is largely seen among women with migraine associated with aura.

(ii) Transdermal Contraceptive Patch (Evra®)

This is a small square adhesive patch to be applied to the skin of the abdomen or buttock. Each patch lasts for seven days and is replaced by a new patch immediately. Each cycle consists of three consecutive weeks of transdermal application and one week of no patch application. The patch delivers to systemic circulation of 20 µg of ethinylestradiol and 150 µg of norelgetromin daily.

Transdermal contraceptive patch has a similar efficacy as the OCP. Compared to OCP users, patch users have better compliance per cycle. But because of the higher incidence of side effects from breast engorgement and tenderness, and nausea and vomiting, patch users have a higher discontinuation rate compared to OCP users.

(iii) Vaginal Contraceptive Ring (NuraRing®)

This is a flexible tubal ring device for vaginal application. It contains ethinylestradiol and etonogestrel, an active derivative of desogestrel. Each ring stays in the vagina for three weeks and is replaced after one week of ring-free interval.

The contraceptive efficacy, compliance and discontinuation rates are similar between vaginal ring and OCP users. The adverse effects are also comparable between the groups, except than more ring users experience vaginal irritation.

(iv) Depot-medroxyprogesterone Acetate (DMPA)

This is a highly effective form of longer-term contraception with three-monthly intramuscular injection of 150 mg medroxyprogesterone acetate. The contraceptive failure rate is 0.2% per year or cumulative failure rate of 0.7% at three years. The access to re-supply by repeated visits has resulted in high discontinue rate of 40% at one year.

It is widely used in lactating women and in adolescents and young women. The return of fertility may take 12–18 months. Long-term use of DMPA is associated with deleterious effects on lipid profile, weight gains, menstrual changes, and osteoporosis.

Its use is contraindicated in women with known risk factors for cardiovascular diseases, hormone sensitive cancers and osteoporosis. DMPA, on the other hand, is associated with reduced pain from endometriosis and sickle cell crisis.

(v) Subcutaneous Implant (Implanon NXT)

This is a long-term reversible contraceptive for a period of three years. The device is a single 4-cm ethylene vinyl acetate rod containing 68 mg of the etonorgestrel. The mode of contraceptive action arises from ovulation inhibition, thickening of cervical mucus which inhibits sperm penetration and possibly preventing implantation by thinning the endometrium. The contraceptive efficacy is 99.9%.

The device is implanted directly under the skin of the upper, inner, non-dominant arm using local anesthetic. After three years, a small skin incision over the device is made to retrieve the rod and a new one can be inserted immediately. Technical difficulty on retrieving the device is encountered in 1% of cases.

The most frequently encountered adverse effect of Implanon NXT is menstrual changes. Approximately three in five women experience infrequent and irregular bleeding, one in five reports amenorrhea, and one in five experiences frequent and prolonged bleeding. There is a reduced pain from endometriosis.

(vi) Intrauterine Device (IUD)

These are highly effective long-term reversible method of contraception for three to five years. There are copper-containing and levonorgestrel-impregnated types of IUD.

Mirena® is a T-shape device impregnated with 52 mg of levonorgestrel which is released at a rate of 20 µg daily over five years. Its contraceptive efficacy is 99.8%. Levonorgestrel induces severe endometrial atrophy, thickening of cervical mucus, and delay in ovulation.

The low systemic delivery of the hormone leads to hardly any systemic progestational effects. However, prolonged scanty vaginal bleeding is common in the initial months of use. Subsequently, the bleeding pattern improves to become either a reduced menstrual flow, infrequent and irregular bleeding, or amenorrhea.

Joydess® is a modified Mirena® with a slimmer device carrying 13.5 mg of levonorgestrel with a daily release of 8 µg for a total of three years. The contraceptive efficacy is 99% and the menstrual changes are less compared to Implanon NXT. The discontinuation rate at 12 months is 10%.

Nova-T380® is a copper containing non-hormonal IUD. Copper ions are toxic to sperm and it induces endometrial changes unfavorable for implantation. It is used for five years with a contraceptive efficacy of 99.2%. The device is associated with increased menstruation and pelvic pain. For an unclear mechanism, copper IUD users have a reduced risk of endometrial and cervical cancers.

(vii) Condoms

These are generally latex condoms, though polyurethane condoms are available for couples allergic to latex. The pregnancy rate approaches 15–20% in a year among couples who use male condom as the sole method of contraception. Condom is an effective contraception for couples in whom the woman has contraindication to other forms of contraception. It is also effective in reducing many types of sexually transmissible infection such as human immunodeficiency virus.

(viii) Permanent Contraception

This is generally a surgical procedure to occlude or to remove part of the fallopian tubes. It is one of the most common methods of contraception in women above 35-years old and in whom cessation of fertility is intended. The prevalence rate of permanent contraception averages 20%, ranging up to 35% in India.

Post-partum tubal ligation. This is done during caesarean section or through a mini-laparotomy at the level of umbilicus within 48 hours of delivery. A partial salpingectomy has a failure rate of approximately 0.6/1000 in one year and 7.5/1000 in 10 years. The use of titanium (Filshie) clips to occlude the isthmus portion of the fallopian tubes appears to have more contraceptive failure as compared with partial salpingectomy (0.017 versus 0.004 over 24 months).

Interval laparoscopic tubal occlusion. This can be achieved with electrocoagulation, mechanical occlusion with silicone rubber bands, spring clips or titanium clips, and partial or total salpingectomy. The procedure is safe but operative complication occurs at a rate of 0.9–1.6 per 100 procedures. The 10-year follow up pregnancy rate is approximately 7.5/1000 procedure.

Total salpingectomy. Recent interest in total salpingectomy as a form of permanent contraception is based on the understanding that some ovarian cancers originate from fimbria cells. The operation duration is longer than partial salpingectomy and is more costly than clip occlusion of the tubes.

Hysteroscopic tubal occlusion. This is an office procedure under local paracervical anesthetic. The procedure involves placing the Essure (USA) devise into the proximal portion of the fallopian tube under hysteroscopic guidance. Essure is the occlusion agent and it consists of a nickel–titanium alloy outer coil and a stainless-steel inner coil wrapped in polyethylene terephthalate fibres. The achievement of complete bilateral tubal occlusion has to be confirmed with a hysterosalpingogram three months after the procedure, during which alternative contraception is needed. The reported success rate is between 76% and 96%.

What is Post-coital Contraception?

Post-coital contraception is also known as emergency contraception. It is used to prevent pregnancy after unprotected sexual intercourse or failure of contraceptive method such as condom breakage or missed doses of oral contraceptives.

(i) **Copper IUD.** This is the most effective emergency contraceptive within five days of sexual intercourse and is not affected by the woman's body weight. The pregnancy rate is 0.1%. It can be carried out as a long-term contraception. The barrier to the use of IUD is availability of trained personnel for its insertion.

(ii) **Ulipristal Acetate (UPA).** This is a selective progesterone receptor modulator (SPRM). Single oral dose at 30 mg delays ovulation, even after LH has started to rise. It is more effective than the levonorgestrel-only (LNG) regimen and maintains its efficacy for up to five days. Repeated use of UPA every five to seven days is safe.

Resumption of non-hormonal contraception can begin immediately after UPA but OCP resumption should begin not sooner than five days after UPA.

(iii) **LNG (Levonorgestrel)**, 1.5 mg, by delaying ovulation before LH surge, is an effective emergency contraception. The pregnancy rate is affected by the woman's body weight: 1.4% for women weighing 65–75 kg and 6.4% for women weighing more than 75 kg.

(iv) **The Yuzpe Regimen**, consisting of two doses of 100 µg of ethinyl estradiol and 0.5–1.0 mg of LNG, is the least effective method and is commonly associated with nausea. It is used when progestin-only emergency contraception is not available.

(v) **Mifepristone** (10–25 mg) is also available as an emergency contraception in China, Russia and Vietnam.

What Options does she have when an Unplanned Pregnancy Occurs?

Unplanned, mistimed and unwanted pregnancies, regardless of the use of contraception, are known collectively as unintended pregnancies. A national survey in USA in 2006–2008 reported that 50% of the pregnancies were unintended. Unintended pregnancies can be stressful. Physicians play an important role in assisting women to reach an informed decision, in a nonjudgmental way and with respect to their decision and rights, and in guiding them to appropriate resources.

Three options are available to women who have an unintended pregnancy:

(i) Continue the Pregnancy to Term and Raising the Child

The outcome of unintended pregnancies is worse than other pregnancies. Compared to other pregnancies, perinatal mortality rate doubles and the rate of extremely low birth weight is five times higher in unintended pregnancies overall. Several reasons have been suggested to explain these observations. Women with unintended pregnancies receive less than the recommended antenatal care such as lower rate of preconception folic acid use, exhibit increased prenatal and postnatal tobacco use, and are less likely to initiate first-trimester prenatal care.

Physicians should direct these women to appropriate obstetric care and resources for social and financial assistance during the pregnancy and after childbirth.

(ii) Continue the Pregnancy to Term and Choosing Adoption

Not many women with unintended pregnancies choose to offer the children for adoption. Factors favoring choosing adoption are women with higher education levels and high career or educational aspirations, women who have had positive personal experiences with adoption, women whose boyfriends or mothers want them to choose adoption, and women who expect little assistance with child care from their mothers.

Physicians may provide information, advice, or prenatal care to these women but must not broker adoptions, match potential parents with mothers, or adopt children of their own patients. Multiple resources and legal agencies are available for women interested in adoption.

(iii) **Induced Abortion**

Women considering an induced abortion should be informed adequately about the potential health risks of abortion and continued pregnancy. With appropriate counseling and legalized skillful medical management, induced abortion is safe and with no long-term emotional or psychological sequelae. There is no significant impact on the woman's subsequent obstetric performance either. It is, in fact, associated with a lower relative risk of obstetric morbidity as pregnancy is often complicated by hypertensive disorders, antepartum and postpartum hemorrhage, and surgical procedure such as cesarean section.

Approximately 50% of unintended pregnancies are terminated by induced abortion, depending on the available abortion law. In Singapore legislature, the gestational age limitation for induced abortion is 24 completed weeks, counting from the first day of the last menstrual period. Singapore legislature further requires the woman to declare her marital status, educational level and number of living children, and to undertake a mandatory counseling by trained personnel. There must be a time lapse of at least 48 hours between professional counseling and the woman's giving the formal consent for induced abortion.

- *Medical-induced abortion.* Pregnancies in the first trimester can undergo induced abortion with Mifepristone (Mifeprex), 600 mg orally, followed by misoprostol (Cytotec), 400 µg orally 48 hours later, or Misoprostol, 800 µg orally or vaginally every three hours for 12 hours. The success rate is 90% and it carries an advantage of avoiding anesthesia and invasive surgical procedure. Complications are rare but include infection, pain that requires analgesia, prolonged vaginal bleeding, and hemorrhage that requires emergency surgery.

Medical-induced abortion for pregnancies in the second trimester is performed with induced labor using mifepristone 200 mg, followed by misopristol 400 µg vaginally or sublingually three-hourly (repeated for up to a maximum of five applications on the same day), or gemeprost 1 mg vaginal pessary every three hours for a maximum of five pessaries in 24 hours. The success rate is more than 80% within 24 hours.

- *Surgical-induced abortion* is done by dilatation and vacuum aspiration and/or curettage. It can be done for pregnancies in the first and second trimesters. Compared to medical-induced abortion, it has a very high success rate and has less blood loss. The procedure completes rapidly and no specific patient follow up is necessary. The disadvantage of surgical method is the need for anesthesia and the risk of cervical and uterine trauma.

Illustration of Some Conditions Related to Contraceptives

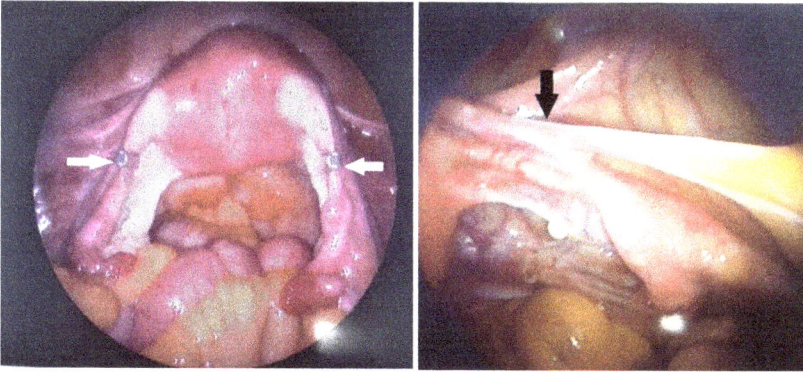

This panel of photographs of laparoscopy shows tubal occlusion with Filshie clips (white arrows on the left panel) and adhesion of bowel to the site of transected portion of the fallopian tube (black arrow on the right panel).

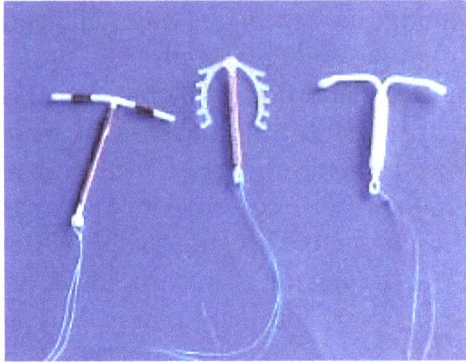

This photograph shows three types of IUD: (from the left): Copper-T, Multiload, and Mirena.

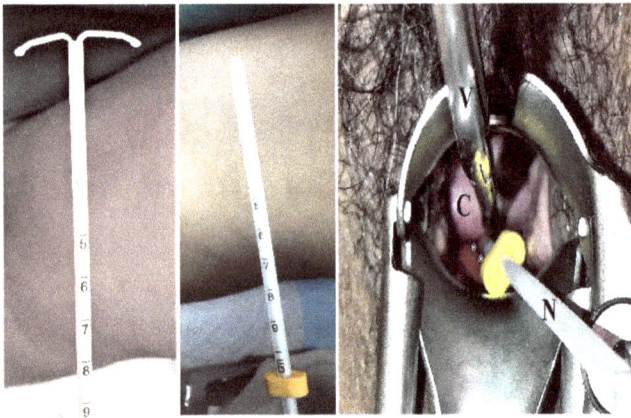

The procedure of insertion of a Nova-T copper IUD is shown in this photograph. The panel on the extreme left shows the device. The middle panel shows that the IUD has been retracted into the insertion sheath (marked by "N" in the extreme right panel). "C" is the cervix held with vulsellum forceps (marked "V") and the IUD device (marked "N") inserted into the uterine cavity via the cervix.

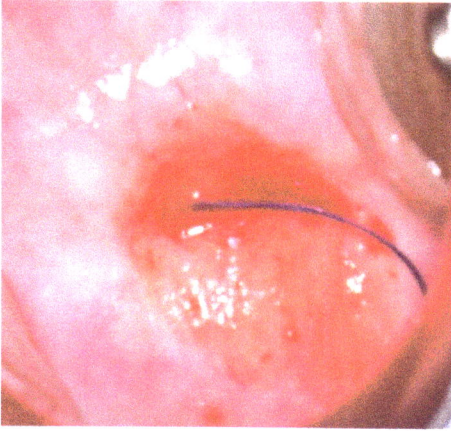

This photograph of the cervix shows a blue string of the IUD. Its presence is assurance of the presence of the IUD and is needed for retrieval of the IUD.

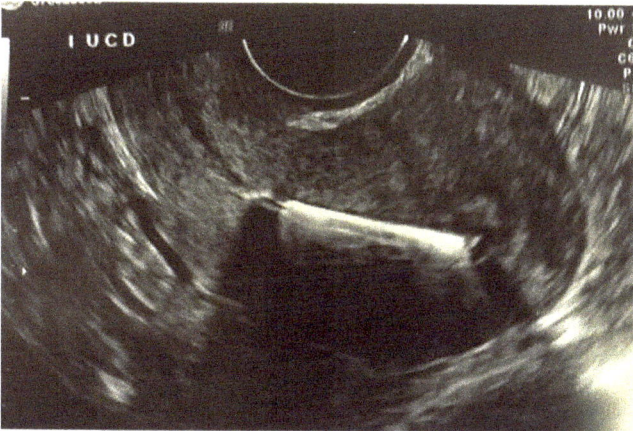

This photograph of an ultrasound scan shows the dense shadow of a copper intrauterine device. (Mirena does not show up clearly on ultrasound scan.)

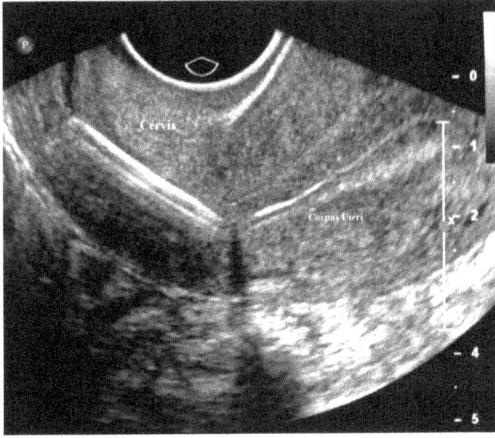

This photograph shows the shadow of the IUD in the cervical canal. It was an IUD that had been partially expulsed.

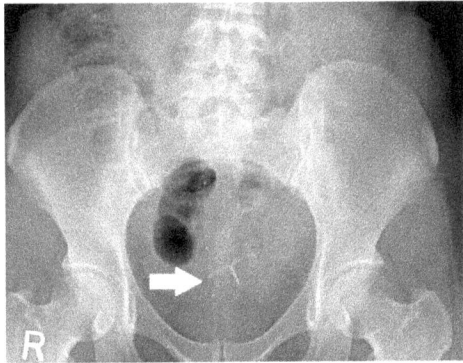

Mirena is radio-opaque (white arrow). as shown in this photograph of a plain X-ray.

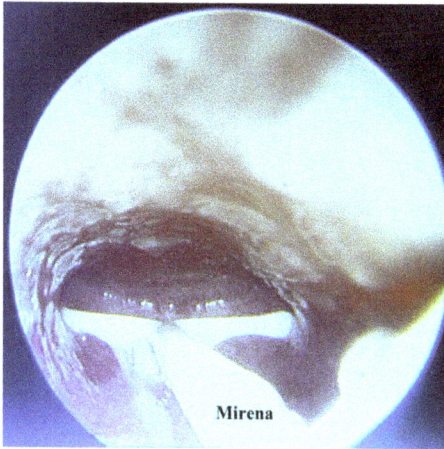

This photograph of a hysteroscopy shows a piece of Mirena in the uterine cavity. Note the severely atrophic endometrium after prolonged use of Mirena.

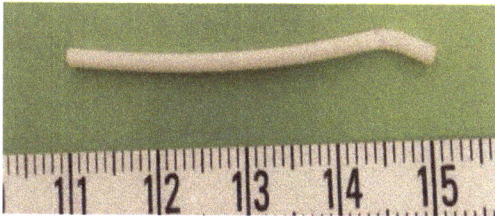

This photograph shows the rod of Implanon retrieved at the end of 3 years.

CASE 23 — HOT FLUSHES

A 50-year-old woman complains of hot flushes and excessive perspiration.

- What is menopause?
- What is menopausal transition?
- What are the major health issues related to menopause?

What is Menopause?

Menopause defines the cessation of reproductive function of a woman by loss of ovarian function either as a result of the aging process or an iatrogenic process, such as bilateral ovariectomy or pelvic irradiation. Premature menopause, now more appropriately termed primary ovarian insufficiency, refers to cessation of ovulation and secretion of estrogen, progesterone and testosterone in young women before the age of 40-years. In clinical practice, menopause is diagnosed when menstruation ceases spontaneously for a period of 12 months consecutively.

During menopause, failure of ovarian follicular development as a consequence of natural follicular atresia results in cessation of ovarian secretion of estradiol, progesterone and testosterone. This is marked by elevation of serum levels of follicle stimulating hormone (FSH) and, to a smaller degree, luteinizing hormone (LH), and a decreased anti-müllerian hormone (AMH). The source of a small quantity of estrogen after menopause is estrone from peripheral aromatization of androstenedione secreted by the adrenal glands and stroma of the ovaries.

Physiological menopause occurs at a mean age of 51.3 years, which has remained unchanged since the known medical history.

The prevalence of menopause between 45- and 55-years old was reported in a large cross-sectional analysis of 2570 women in 1992 from the Massachusetts Women's Health Study:

Age (yr)	Prevalence of Menopause (%)
45	8
46	9
47	14
48	20
49	27
50	36
51	46
52	58
53	70
54	78
55	82

What is Menopausal Transition?

Menopausal transition, previously termed climacteric or perimenopause, is a period of time when symptoms of declining ovarian functions begin to manifest clinically. It lasts five to six years and, typically has the onset between 45 and 47 years and may include the immediate postmenopausal years. During the early phase of the menopausal transition, ovarian resistance to FSH stimulation occurs as the pool of available oocytes for recruitment each cycle diminishes and, increasingly, more cycles are anovulatory. However, once a follicle develops and ovulation occurs, the luteal phase remains normal and pregnancy is possible. Elevation of serum FSH level is indicative of menopausal transition, but the wide biological range of serum FSH levels makes a single FSH value uninformative clinically. A rising trend in serial serum FSH determination is the biochemical hallmark of menopausal transition but its clinical utility is unnecessary.

Clinical Symptoms of Menopausal Transition

More than 95% of women experience at least one symptom during menopausal transition. The prevalence of symptoms reaches a peak at 47-years and declines in the ensuing five years for breast tenderness, palpitations, dizziness, irritability, anxiety or depression, tearfulness, and frequent severe headaches. In contrast, the prevalence of insomnia, musculoskeletal aches and joint pain, hot flushes, vaginal dryness, and difficulties with sexual intercourse increases between the age of 48 and 54 years. Of all the symptoms, insomnia, irritability/anxiety, severe hot flushes and sweating, and vaginal dryness carry the highest negative impact on the quality of life.

- *Irregular menstruation.* The most characteristic change of menstruation during menopausal transition is a short menstrual cycle of less than 25 days in duration. This is the result of increasing unresponsiveness of ovaries to FSH stimulation. Other types of abnormal uterine bleeding require further evaluation to exclude endometrial or intrauterine pathology.
- *Hot flushes*: Hot flushes occur in 75% of women during menopausal transition. These are brief experience of a sudden onset of sensation of warmth, most commonly in the face (78%), neck (74%) and chest (61%). In some women, hot flushes spread throughout the entire body. It may be associated with redness in the face as in blushes. Hot flushes can occur during day or night and is often accompanied by sweating and/or palpitation. According to women's self-reported rating, the severity of hot flushes shows a prevalence distribution of mild in 41%, moderate in 43%, severe in 13% and very severe in 1.8%. Similarly, the prevalence of bothersome flushes is mild in 43%, moderate in 33%, severe in 17.5% and very bothersome in 6%. The duration of this symptom shows a wide variation between individual women. The median duration of hot flushes is one year. In women with moderate to severe flushes, the median duration may last for five years, and one third of

these women report the symptoms for 10 years or more after the final menstruation period.

- *Insomnia*. Sleep disorder, defined by the Athens Insomnia Scale (AIS) in a self-administered psychometric instrument designed for quantifying sleep difficulty, is found in 40% among women aged 40–44 years and in 45% among those aged 55–59 years. Day dysfunction (sleepiness) was most commonly observed among women in the menopausal transition period and less commonly among late postmenopausal women. A strong relationship exists between insomnia and anxiety and depression, use of hypnotic drugs, presence of vasomotor symptoms and alcoholism.

  Sleep disorder of menopausal transition seems to be related to low progesterone rather than estrogen. Progesterone has sedative and anxiolytic properties by increasing the effectiveness of γ-aminobutyric acid (GABA). Experience of estrogen replacement therapy alone has not shown a consistent improvement on insomnia.

- *Anxiety and depression*. Mood changes and mental irritability are often reported by women in the menopausal transition years. In a long-term Zurich community-based study, it was reported that the 12-month prevalence rate of major depressive episode was 18.5% among premenopausal women, 13.8% among menopausal transition women, and 11.1% among postmenopausal women. A similar 12-month prevalence rate of 22% to 24% for anxiety disorders were reported for women in these three categories of menopausal status. There is a strong association between mood disorders during menopausal transition and psychiatric disorders during the younger years. Current evidence support the notion that anxiety disorders and depression during menopausal transition is related to life events and prior psychiatric disorders than sex hormone deficiency of menopause.

- *Fatigue, tiredness and lack of energy*. These symptoms, when overwhelming, are associated with impairment of physical and cognitive functions. It is important to exclude specific underlying medical disorders, including thyroid disease, anemia, adrenal insufficiency and sequelae of history of stroke and cardiac diseases.

These symptoms are reported in 50% of women during menopausal transition. In the great majority of cases, the complaints are either a consequence of sleep disorder or are related to stress, anxiety, depression or other psychological condition.

- *Low or loss of libido.* Large community-based 10-year follow-up of women, aged 42–52-years old, reported that the prevalence of having sexual desire once or more per week declined from 58.4% at baseline to 35% at year-10. However, there were no discernible changes in frequency of sexual arousal and orgasm. Estrogen has not been found to play a role in any of these domains of sexual function. Evidence for the role of androgen in female sexual function is conflicting. Blood circulating level of androgen declines with age, which includes menopausal transition years, but no diagnostic cut-off level of androgen is currently available for clinical definition of androgen deficiency in women. Furthermore, women's sexual desire is conditional to a complex process of physical, emotional and sociopsychological states. The declining libido in women is, therefore, to be treated as more of an age-related change than hormonal fluctuation of menopausal transition.

- *Vaginal dryness.* Vaginal dryness during menopausal transition is reported as mild in 70%, moderately severe in 12%, and very severe in 7% of women. Another 10% of women experiences severe vaginal dryness late in the menopause years.

- *Musculoskeletal ache and pain.* Nearly 50% of middle age women reports pain and joint stiffness. The prevalence of these symptoms shows a rising trend across the years of menopausal transition. Multifactorial analysis indicates that the symptoms are associated with high body mass index, negative mood and radiological diagnosis of osteoarthritis.

- *Headache, dizziness and vertigo.* Headache is reported in 16% and dizziness and/or vertigo in 30% of women during menopausal transition. In general, women of reproductive age experience more migraine than men, in a ratio of 3:1, and the prevalence reaches a peak at 42-years old. The neural hyper-responsive effects of estrogen are mediated via glutaminergic, serotonergic, opiatergic and noradrenergic systems. In contrast, progesterone and its metabolite induce a hypo-responsive neural effect through activation of GABAnergic system and modulation of estrogenic effects in the central nervous system. Rapid decline in estrogen and progesterone in the late luteal phase is a triggering factor for migraine in some women. Migraine without aura, compared to migraine with aura, is particularly sensitive to ovarian hormone fluctuations. It is recently recognized that there is a form of vestibular migraine characterized by a highly variable temporal relationship between migraine and vestibular symptoms of dizziness and/or vertigo. It is most probable that the common complaints of headache, dizziness and/or vertigo during menopausal transition are caused by vestibular migraine triggered by fluctuation of estrogen and progesterone during this period of time.

What are the Major Health Issues related to Menopause?

Menopause-related Disorders

Women in developed countries spend a third or more of their lifespan in the state of menopause. Menopausal health issues are medical conditions in which the onset and disease progression are significantly influenced by withdrawal of ovarian hormones. They carry a negative impact on quality of life and morbidity and mortality of these women.

(i) *Osteoporosis*

Physiological bone turnover is a balance of osteoblast and osteoclast activities. Estrogen exerts an important physiological role in bone physiology via estrogen receptor-β on these cells. During menopause, there is an exaggerated rate of bone loss which affects trabecular bone more than cortical bone. It is estimated that, of the total bone loss, almost 50% occurs in the first 5–10 years of menopause.

Bone mass is directly correlated to the tensile strength of the bone. Reducing bone mass increases the rate of bone fractures. Currently, clinical estimation of risk of bone fracture is measured by bone mineral density (BMD) by means of dual-energy X-ray absorptiometry (DXA). Using the peak BMD as a reference, a measurement of negative 1–2.49 standard deviations is termed osteopenia. Osteoporosis is defined by a BMD measurement of negative 2.5 standard deviations or more below the reference range.

In Singapore, the prevalence of osteoporosis of the spine and head of femurs in menopausal women is 6.5% and 23.4%, respectively, as compared with 0.5% and 7.1%, respectively, among premenopausal women. For women between 51- and 60-years of age, and who are not on estrogen replacement therapy, the prevalence of spine and femoral osteoporosis is 3.8% and 15.7%, respectively. The prevalence rate increases in women above 60-years old to 10.5% and 36.8%, respectively. Among women on estrogen-containing hormone replacement therapy, the rate of osteoporosis is approximately 2.5% for the spine and 14% for the femur.

The rate of osteoporotic fracture markedly increases from 4% in women between 50- and 59-years old to 52% for women above 80-years old. It is interesting to note that the pattern of fractures changes during the menopausal years, with fracture of the lower end of radius bone in the first decade, fracture of the vertebrae in the second decade, and fracture of the femoral hip in later years.

(ii) *Cardiovascular Diseases*

The risk of cardiovascular diseases (CVD) increases with age for both men and women, with the incidence of CVD among women lagging behind men by 10 years. The gap of difference by gender, however, diminishes with increasing age because of higher rate of increase in CVD in women compared to men. Statistics from the American Heart Association (2007) showed that the rate of increase in the incidence of CVD was similar among men and women for the decade from 45–54-years old to 55–64-years old (110%). But the rate of increase doubled in women (124%) as compared with men (61%) for the decade from 55–64-years old to 65–74-years old.

The link of menopause to CVD is also provided by observations that women who have more total menstruation years exhibit a lower risk of CVD compared to their counterparts.

Menopause is a state of relative predominance of bioavailable testosterone as a result of the diminishing circulatory levels of estrogen and sex-hormone binding globulin. This, in turn, is associated with a rapid progression in the severity of metabolic syndrome, visceral obesity, and secretion of pro-inflammatory cytokines. These pathophysiological changes are risk factors for CVD.

(iii) *Menopausal Genitourinary Syndrome*

Menopausal genitourinary syndrome refers to a set of symptoms related to changes in the vulva, vagina, bladder and urethra as a consequence of loss of endogenous estrogen. The syndrome affects approximately 30% of menopausal women, of which 60% actively seeks medical treatment. The presenting symptoms include pruritus vulvae, vulvodynia, dyspareunia, loss of libido and poor sexual responses, apareunia, post-coital bleeding, vaginal discharge or staining of blood, frequency and urgency of micturition, dysuria and urinary incontinence. The severity of individual symptoms varies between affected women and, by the predominance of the presenting symptoms, the condition has variously been termed atrophic vulvovaginitis, atrophic vaginitis, overactive bladder, and others.

Clinically, menopausal vulvar atrophy appears pale in color and flattened in contour. The introitus appears narrow. The pubic hair is sparse. The vaginal mucosa is smooth from loss of rugae and may show petechia or epithelial ulcerations.

Embryologically, the lower urinary and genital tracts developed from the same primitive urogenital sinus. These structures are highly sensitive to estrogenic influences throughout the entire life of a woman. Loss of estrogen results in epithelial atrophy in the vagina, vestibular mucosa, and trigon region of the urinary bladder and other urothelium. The diminished peri-vaginal and peri-urethral collagen leads to anatomical shrinkage from loss of tissue turgor and elasticity. Loss of estrogen also reduces the vaginal epithelial glycogen production which leads to diminished population of lactobacilli and a rising vaginal fluid pH value. These environmental changes facilitate vaginal colonization of fecal flora and bacteriuria.

The mainstay treatment of menopausal genitourinary syndrome is topical estrogen therapy. Intra-vaginal estrogen therapy, either in the form of cream, pessary or vagina ring, has been shown to be effective in improving vaginal dryness and lubrication and in reducing dyspareunia. It has been reported that the serum estradiol level of vaginal estrogen therapy is one-fourth of oral estrogen therapy but with a four-fold higher potency. Continual treatment is needed to prevent vulvovaginal atrophy and long-term vaginal therapy is safe with an extremely low risk of endometrial hyperplasia.

Therapy with vaginal moisturizers or lubricants reduces vaginal dryness but does not alleviate symptoms from loss of vaginal elasticity and dyspareunia from thin vagina.

Vaginal estrogen therapy has also been shown to improve the irritating urinary symptoms of frequency and urgency symptoms, and in urge incontinence of urine when used in conjunction with anticholinergic medications.

(iv) Alzheimer's Disease and Dementia

The prevalence of Alzheimer's disease (AD) and dementia increases with age, with a significant gender difference. At 90-years old, the prevalence of AD is 3.4 times higher among women compared to men. In contrast, vascular dementia remains similar between the genders. The cumulative risk of AD from 65-years old to 90-years old was 2.5 times higher for women (0.22) compared to men (0.09).

However, in a meta-analysis of available publications in 2016, it was found that age at menopause was not associated with AD and dementia collectively (1.16, 95% CI: 0.74, 1.83). Also, it was not associated with dementia from all causes excluding AD (0.96, 95% CI: 0.78, 1.21). Currently, the role of withdrawal of sex hormone steroidal neuro-regulations during menopause in the observed excess risk of AD in women remains unproven.

Illustration of Some Conditions Associated with Menopause

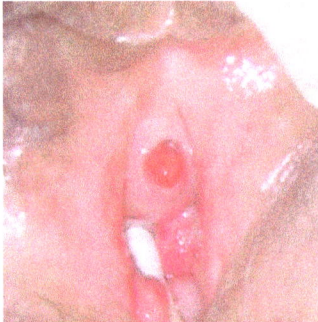

This elderly woman complained of recurrent urinary frequency and urgency. This photograph shows atrophic changes of thinning in the mucosa of the introitus and a red mass protruding out of the urethral meatus. This lesion was prolapsed urethral mucosa from the eversion of the meatus as the result of loss of peri-urethral submucosal collagen tissue. The lesion is sometimes called urethral caruncle. The condition resolves on topical estrogen therapy.

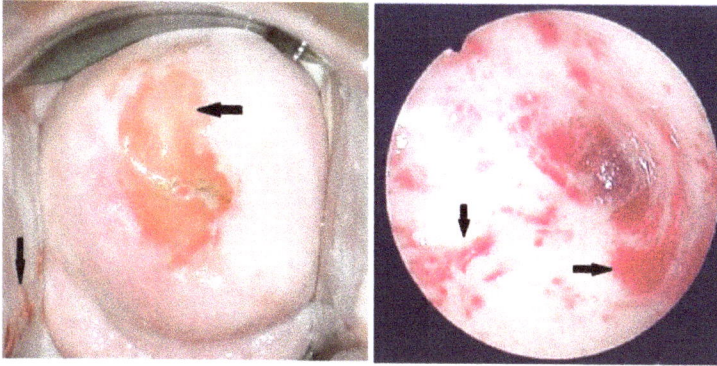

This panel of photographs shows the appearance of menopausal atrophy of the endometrium, the cervix and vagina. The thin epithelium of these structures appears pale in color and the underlying vascular bed appears as patches of redness (marked by arrows).

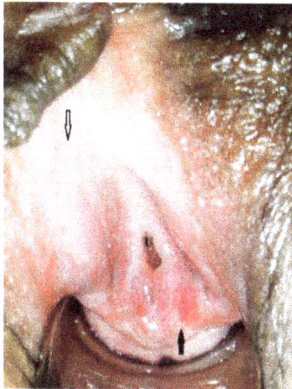

This menopausal woman complained of a dull discomfort in the vagina. The photograph shows atrophic changes in the vulva with thin and pale mucosa (marked by open arrow) and capillary bed visible from the thin and transparent mucosa (solid arrow). The urethral meatus is marked "U".

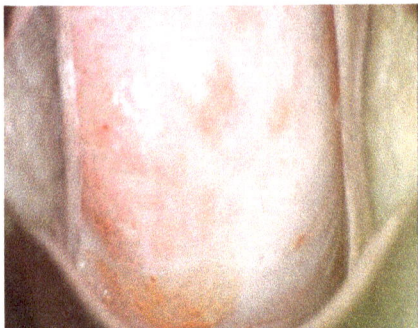

This photograph shows menopausal atrophy of the vagina. The mucosa is pale in color and smooth with loss of rugae.

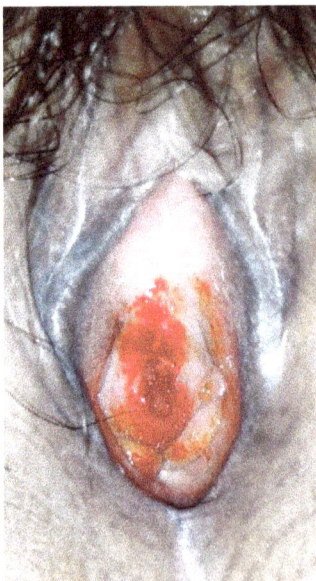

This elderly woman complained of pink-color staining on the undergarment. The photograph shows severe atrophy of the mucosa with hemorrhagic appearance at the introitus.

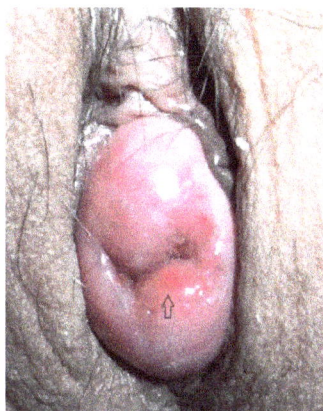

This menopausal woman presented with a lump down below. The lump was the cervix of the uterus as shown in this photograph. This was a grade-2 prolapse of the uterus from menopausal degenerative atrophy of the support system of the uterus. The mucosa changes (marked by arrow) of the protruded cervix may lead to ulceration and infection.

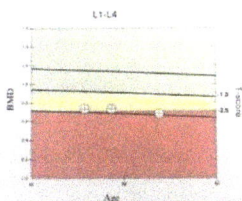

This photograph of a report charting the progressive decline in bone density of lumbar spines measured on dual X-ray densitometry over 4 years. In 2008, the T-score fell below the threshold of –2.5 standard deviations and established the clinical diagnosis of osteoporosis by the criteria of the World Health Organization.

INDEX

postmenopausal complex or solid
  cysts, 200
postmenopausal simple cyst, 199
post-partum tubal ligation, 287
post-radiation, 109
premature ovarian failure, 23
premenopausal complex or solid
  cysts, 199
premenopausal simple cyst, 198
premenstrual syndrome, 111
primary amenorrhea, 1
primary dysmenorrhea, 85
procidentia, 151, 154
prolapsed urethral meatus
  mucosa, 78
prostaglandin synthetase
  inhibitors, 53
provoked localized
  vestibule-vulvodynia, 101
pruritus vulvae, 127
psoas abscess, 196
punctation, 255

Q
qualitative PCR-based tests, 118

R
radical hysterectomy, 253
radical trachelectomy, 253
rectocoele, 153
recurrent cystitis, 214
reproductive physiology for
  pregnancy, 268
retention cyst, 105
retrograde menstruation, 96
rhabdomyosarcoma, 251
risk of malignancy index, 230

S
sacrocolpopexy, 151
sacrospinous ligament fixation,
  152
salpingectomy, 268
salpingotomy, 184
SCJ, 65
secondary amenorrhea, 19
secondary dysmenorrhea, 85
segmental salpingectomy, 184
septated uterus, 187
sexually transmitted infections,
  116
Sheehan syndrome, 20
side effects of OCP, 283
skene gland, 158
spontaneous abortion, 186
squamo-columnar junction, 65
squamous cell carcinoma,
  130–132, 139, 142, 243, 251, 254
squamous metaplasia, 65
Stein and Leventhal, 13
stenosis, 26
stress test, 163
subfertility, 13, 22, 90, 92, 223,
  267–271, 276, 277
superficial dyspareunia, 105
surgical induced abortion, 291

T
tamoxifen therapy, 71
telangiectasia, 109
testicular feminization syndrome, 3
Theca-lutein cysts, 193
thelarche, 1
threatened miscarriage, 188
thrombocytopenia, 51

www.ingramcontent.com/pod-product-compliance
Lightning Source LLC
Chambersburg PA
CBHW050540190326
41458CB00007B/1855